WE'VE GOT THIS

Eliza Hull is a contemporary musician, disability advocate, and writer based in regional Victoria, Australia. She has been published in *Growing Up Disabled in Australia* and has a children's book titled *Come Over To My House*. Her music has been used in TV and film, and she was awarded the Arts Access Australia National Leadership Award, the Women in Music Award, and the Music Victoria Award in 2021.

WE'VE

ESSAYS BY

GOT

DISABLED PARENTS

THIS

EDITED BY ELIZA HULL

SCRIBE

Melbourne • London

Scribe Publications
2 John St, Clerkenwell, London, WC1N 2ES, United Kingdom
3754 Pleasant Ave, Suite 100, Minneapolis, Minnesota 55409, USA

Published by arrangement with Black Inc.

Published by Scribe 2023

Typeset in Fournier by Scribe

Printed and bound in the UK by CPI Group (UK) Ltd, Croydon CR0 4YY

Scribe is committed to the sustainable use of natural resources and the use of
paper products made responsibly from those resources.

978 1 957363 25 7 (US edition)
978 1 914484 66 7 (UK edition)
978 1 922586 96 4 (ebook)

Catalogue records for this book are available from the British Library.

scribepublications.com
scribepublications.co.uk

Contents

Introduction

by Eliza Hull

Being a disabled parent is a rebellious act. Disabled people should have the same right to parent as anyone else, but often when we decide to start a family we are met with judgement and discrimination. We are questioned rather than supported. We have to push up against the medical system, which is particularly problematic for disabled people. And we have to confront how ableist society's model of parenting is, even in the twenty-first century. Yet, despite all this, we still choose to parent. And we are damn good at it too!

I became a parent seven years ago. I'd always had an innate drive to have a family. As a child, I wrote in my diary that one day I would become a mother. My parents always hoped I'd have children. When I told them about my desire to be a mother, not once did they discourage the idea; they were excited and supportive of me starting my own family one day.

I have a physical disability, a neurological condition called Charcot-Marie-Tooth. It affects the way I walk. I fall

1

over regularly and have muscle and sensation loss throughout my body. Lack of circulation creates freezing cold legs on hot summer days, and I am consistently fatigued and in pain.

When I first seriously considered having children, I spoke to my neurologist. I had the hugest smile on my face: at the time I was in love and elated just thinking about the possibility of children. I'll never forget his stern and unforgiving look in response; he couldn't hide his disapproval. Silently he wrote notes on his computer as I waited. After what felt like hours, he lifted his head, adjusted his glasses and began to flood me with questions. 'Have you considered your options? As someone with Charcot-Marie-Tooth, you have a 50 per cent chance of passing on your condition. Have you looked into genetic counselling? We could do a panel blood test again? Do you think you will be able to manage?'

I felt like I was crumbling. Shame overcame me. We're taught to trust medical professionals, so his words really stung. I'm used to discrimination: I've had people stop in the street and pray for me. I've been stared at and ridiculed. But this was far more insidious: this was someone in a position of authority, someone who I was supposed to trust, suggesting it would be best if I didn't have a child in case they were *like me*. It affected me deeply. I can still feel the pain in my chest from that day; it flares again in moments of self-doubt.

In June 2014, we found out I was pregnant. A rush of adrenaline filled my body and I had a rollercoaster of emotions: fear, uncertainty and excitement. The neurologist's questions haunted me: how was I going to do this? I grappled with other questions too. Would the pregnancy be too hard on my body? Would people judge me? Could I manage? What if I fell over while holding my baby? At times my head was a whirlwind of anxiety.

I spent hours searching bookshops for a volume about parenting with disability. I wanted to feel represented, read a story like mine, know it was possible. I needed reassurance, to find a friend on the page saying, 'Yes, you can do this.' But there was nothing out there. In all the stacks of parenting books, there were no mums like me. I felt incredibly alone.

Where were the disabled parents? Why couldn't I think of any movie or TV show that included a parent with a disability? In Australia, where I live, more than 15 per cent of households have at least one parent with disability. In the United Kingdom, there are more than 1.7 million disabled parents, while in the United States more than 4.8 million households have a parent with disability. Even though these statistics are so high, we are represented nowhere.

I knew representation mattered – so it became my mission to share the stories of disabled parents, to help other disabled people know they're not alone, and to show it's possible. I searched for other disabled people worldwide who were parents, and little by little I felt less isolated. It became an obsession, and I created a pool of people who I could reach out to. It began to feel like a community of sorts, a way for us all to feel connected. The common thread was that we all felt underrepresented and alone in our decision to parent.

This led me to create the audio series *We've Got This* with the Australian Broadcasting Corporation (ABC). For the series, I travelled around Australia sharing the perspectives of disabled parents. Time and time again, I witnessed that families with disabled parents are just like any other family. Of course they grapple with physical and attitudinal barriers in society, but in their homes all the families I met were thriving.

The thing is, when you're disabled you have to constantly adapt. On a daily basis I have to find unique, creative ways to get around barriers so that I can navigate the world freely. Parenting demands the same kind of innovation. You have to adapt, find solutions, learn about your baby and be constantly flexible.

All new parents know the feeling of bringing your baby home and wondering: *how the hell do I do this?* Disabled parents have an added layer of pressure. Often we feel judged and misunderstood, like the world is watching and waiting for us to make a mistake. Yet because we are already masters at problem solving in daily life, we are perfectly placed to master the art of parenting.

Within this book you will meet parents who identify in a variety of ways. Some parents identify as d/Deaf, disabled, neurodiverse, or chronically ill. Some prefer to call themselves 'disabled'; others prefer 'person with a disability'. My decision to use the subtitle '*essays by disabled parents*' was one I didn't take lightly. In the end, I chose to put our collective disabled identity first: I wanted to express pride and reduce the stigma that we as disabled people continue to face.

Personally, I identify as both a 'disabled parent' and as a 'parent with disability'. I constantly switch back and forth.

Recently I have begun to say 'disabled parent' a lot more and have realised that any discomfort I have ever had with this is my own internalised ableism, stemming from the messages I have continually been fed that disability is a deficit.

The parents who share their stories in *We've Got This* are ingenious, creative and adaptive; they constantly have to navigate physical, attitudinal and social barriers within society. They have faced discrimination and they have had their choice and ability to parent questioned. This is especially the case for parents with intellectual disability. What these parents show us, though, is that parenting isn't black and white. There shouldn't be a template we all follow to the letter. Parenting as disabled people demands we let go of the 'standard' or 'right' way to do something; instead, it's about being creative and flexible – and children are so beautifully open to being adaptive. These stories show us all how rigid the conventional 'template' of parenting is, and these parents display an inner strength that any parent would envy and could learn from.

How do parents who are blind push a pram or measure the right mix of formula and hot water? How do parents who are Deaf know their baby is crying in the night? How does a mother who's a wheelchair user get her baby in and out of the cot, or out of the car? Ultimately, it's always about thinking outside the box.

Throughout my parenting journey, I've learnt ways to be adaptive and innovative. I'm now a mother of two; I have a seven-year-old girl, Isobel, and a two-year-old boy, Archie. At the moment I'm in a world of sleepless nights, pushing prams, and going to storytime at the library.

When Archie was a baby, in the stillness of the night, I would run my hand along the cot, gripping each bar to lead me to the nursing chair, as I held him in the other arm. I grasped the cot tightly as I nestled him in my arms. Every movement was calculated. My senses were alive as I navigated my wobbly, unsteady legs. I had five pillows stacked on the chair to sit on, so I could get myself up while holding a sleeping Archie.

As I slowly moved towards the cot after feeding him, I wondered what it feels like to be held by me. I smile thinking that perhaps the way I moved, the rocking back and forth as I walked, is part of what soothed him to sleep.

Being pregnant the second time was no easier than the first. When you're disabled, you're constantly told by medical professionals and society at large that you ought to be fixed or 'cured'. This fed into a belief that my body was weak, breakable and incompetent. For the whole pregnancy I was riddled with fear that I would lose them, that my body was not stable enough to house a baby. Because of my disability, I also regularly fall over, so this added extra stress. During both pregnancies I visited the maternity ward regularly so I could have the baby's heart rate checked: sometimes after a fall, other times just because I was anxious.

Archie is now a bubbly toddler. He is very different to my daughter. He is a firecracker, full of energy and charisma. At two years old, he loves to run, so I have found it challenging to take him outside the house. When I take him to the park, I go with friends or my partner, who I can rely on to chase him if needed, or I contain him in a little trike that I push and he can't get out of, which my in-laws gave us as a present. Luckily he loves being in it, and it's a wonderful way for me to stabilise as I walk, similar to pushing a walking frame.

At a regular check-up when I was pregnant with Archie, as soon as I waddled in with my large pregnant belly, the obstetrician said, 'I'm hoping you're not going to do this again to yourself: no more for you.' In what world is this appropriate? I should have said something, but I was shocked, so I bit my lip and shrugged it off. What I wanted to say is: how dare you make assumptions, because I'm disabled, about what I choose to do with my body. Instead, the same feeling I'd had when my neurologist questioned me sank in again. The shame washed over me and the immense pain kicked in, causing my heart to feel heavy.

It happened again when I was having an ultrasound. The sonographer asked if I could pass on my disability. I said, 'Yes, there's a 50 per cent chance.' Her mouth dropped open like a fish, before she said, 'Okay, let's see if we can see anything wrong.' I gulped. In that moment, I thought, 'There's nothing wrong with me' – but I couldn't say it aloud.

I have to be honest: having a 50 per cent chance of passing on my genetic condition is not something that's been easy to grapple with. I am proudly disabled, yet I have still worried for my children. I know what kind of world they are coming into; if they have my disability, they will face discrimination, barriers and physical pain, among other societal challenges. This knowledge is hard to navigate.

People may judge me for choosing to parent while knowing

this, but who better to make this decision than someone who's lived with my disability for decades? I am proud of who I am and wouldn't change a thing about me; I want to instil the same pride in my children. I want them to know that whoever they are, it's okay.

The thing is, it's not my disability that disables me: it's society. Being a parent affirmed this for me. As soon as I had kids in tow, I noticed the stares get longer. People began to ask more intrusive questions: What happened to you? What's wrong with you?

When Archie was still little and I needed to get him out of the car, I would lean up against it to steady my legs. I pushed against the car in a squat position with the weight of my body as I slowly manoeuvred him out: everything was done with utmost care and concentration. Yet I always got stared at when I did this.

One day I was pushing Archie in the pram up a slight incline. A man yelled out at the top of his lungs, 'Are you okay? Are you in trouble?' It shocked me. Of course, he may just have been wondering if I was going to make it to the top. Perhaps he was just a caring person, unaware that his comment could be construed as offensive. Or maybe he genuinely wanted to help? But such intrusions never get easier. As other disabled people do, I ask for help when I need it; this felt like an invasion of privacy when I was just going about my day.

Once, when my daughter was eighteen months old, she fell over in the street and I couldn't pick her up because if I did I would lose my balance and fall. People stared at us, wondering why I wasn't lifting her up and soothing her. One lady said,

'Gosh, can you pick her up?' Such judgements hurt. I'll never get used to it, but as I've become more and more proud of my disability identity it affects me less.

Having children was the catalyst for me embracing disability pride. When I first became pregnant, I was still grappling with internalised ableism. I am not even sure I used the word 'disabled' to refer to myself before that. Having children has enabled me to embrace my authentic self. If I'm not proud of who I am, then what is that modelling for my children? I knew if I wanted my children to be proud of who they are, I had to be proud of who I am.

Now Isobel knows my limitations. She's a beautiful child who knows all about disability. She will move toys on the floor in the house out of the way so that I have a path to walk along without falling over. I love the feeling of her hand in mine as we cross the road; she will often hold it extra tightly in case I fall. Sometimes she will help pull me across the road so we make it while the lights are red. The first time she noticed I had a disability, she said, 'Mum, why do you always walk like a penguin?' How innocent and sweet. We laughed and laughed together about it.

One day, when we were in the line to get into preschool, a child from her class asked, 'Why do you walk like that?' The mother first tried to shush her child, then she looked at me and back at her child and said, 'She's been in an accident.' She knew it wasn't true. She knew I was disabled, and not from an accident, but obviously to her this explanation was too hard, the word 'disabled' too daunting for her to tackle. As we moved away from them into the kinder room, my daughter looked up and said, 'You're disabled, Mum' and smiled knowingly.

I take immense joy in knowing that my kids have this sense of pride. They are part of a diverse family where disability is celebrated and accepted – not something to be feared. Now, when asked, my daughter always says proudly, 'My mum has a disability.' This is one of the many positives of being a disabled parent: seeing compassion, kindness and openness to all differences grow in our children. Ultimately this builds a more inclusive society for everyone – after all, our kids are the future.

One of the biggest barriers that parents with disability face, especially parents with intellectual disability, is lack of support. Often we expect parents to be autonomous, to parent alone without the required supports and education. In many countries in the Western world including Australia, the United Kingdom and the United States, up to 80 per cent of parents with intellectual disability will have their kids removed. This is mostly due to these parents not being given the chance to learn, or adequate support so that they can keep their children in their care. Often children of parents with intellectual disability are portrayed as victims and parents are seen as incompetent and are infantilised. Yet if given the required supports, parents with intellectual disability make incredible parents. The grief for parents with intellectual disability when they are separated from their children has a profound impact on their health and wellbeing and that of their children. My hope for the future is that we can put more in place to support parents with intellectual disability to keep their children in their care. This would need to be a safe, non-judgemental support system that doesn't set these parents up to fail.

Another barrier to parenting as a disabled person is involuntary, non-therapeutic sterilisation, which has been carried out in Australia since the 1800s. Unbelievably, coercive or forced sterilisation is still an ongoing practice in Australia, often occurring under a pretext of being in the person's 'best interests'. Disabled people, especially women and girls, are still having their choice to parent stolen from them. The exact number of sterilisations being carried out is unknown, but may be increasing. In the United States of America, most states allow forced sterilisation today. Laws allowing forced sterilisation exist in thirty-one states as well as Washington, DC. In Canada in 1986, the Supreme Court ruled that disabled people could not be sterilised without their consent, yet it continues to take place, often disguised using medical reasons, while long-term contraceptives are recommended at a higher rate, without explaining their impact on preventing pregnancy.

In 2012, an Australian Human Rights Commission report noted that while 'the authorisation of either the Family Court of Australia or a state or territory guardianship tribunal is required before a child or adult with disability can be involuntarily sterilised (except in emergency situations in which there is a serious threat to life or health)', the legal and regulatory frameworks and guidelines 'have failed to protect women and girls with disability from involuntary or coerced sterilisation'.

Disabled people shouldn't be denied the right to parent. Yet it's still common for people to hold entrenched assumptions about what disabled people can and can't do, and therefore lose control of their own choices about their body and decision to parent.

Yet despite all these obstacles, there are so many disabled people parenting successfully. Some of their stories are shared in this book. Each experience is unique, and some intersect with other identities: *We've Got This* includes parents who are queer, nonbinary, Indigenous or from Culturally and Linguistically Diverse backgrounds. Some contributors wrote their own pieces; I wrote up other people's stories from interviews. While the experiences captured are enormously diverse, they share some common themes – and all parents were candid in sharing the challenges and, yes, joys in parenting with disability.

In sharing their stories, I hope to counter some of the myths and misconceptions surrounding disabled parents.

Of course, being a disabled parent is not easy. There are times when I wish I had more energy or wasn't in pain – when I'm pushing the pram around the block and my bones feel like glass, sharp pain like razor blades shoots around my body. But then I look inside the pram and see a smiling face, and it's all worth it. There are moments that hurt: when my partner is running around with the kids or is able to hold them and carry them in ways I can't and never will. Or the pinch in my chest when I see other mothers 'baby wearing' with their child in a sling or carrier, when this was never a possibility for me. But I know I'm an incredible mother. My daughter and I paint and read together. I sit on the ground and roll the ball up and down with my energetic son. But most significantly, I'm teaching them the importance of a diverse and inclusive world. I don't parent despite my disability; I parent as a proudly disabled person. Being a disabled parent is not a deficit; we create a rich, colourful life where difference is celebrated and embraced.

Parenting with a disability doesn't look like following a textbook; it looks like love, connection, pride, innovation and adaptability. We're rebellious, not in a brave, heroic way – more in a bad-arse way! We face so many societal barriers as soon as we decide to parent. I hope by the time you have finished this book, you'll agree with me that it shouldn't be this way. I also hope that we will begin to experience a more inclusive world where being a disabled parent is accepted and normalised – where it is no longer a rebellious act, but just another form of parenting.

I hope that all readers – disabled or not, parents or not – will find something empowering about reading these stories of resistance and rebellion, courage and creativity.

And for any disabled person about to dive into the unknown, exciting, terrifying and heart-exploding world of parenting, I want you to know there's a community of people out there to support you – you're not alone. I hope this book will help you realise that – like all the parents who share their stories here – *you've got this!*

* * *

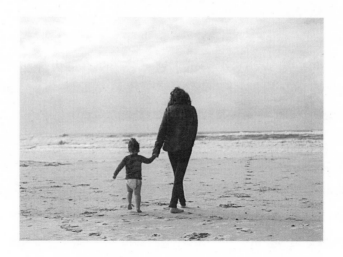

Eliza Hull is a contemporary musician, disability advocate and writer based in regional Victoria. She has been published in *Growing Up Disabled in Australia* and her podcast series on parenting with a disability, *We've Got This*, was one of Radio National's and ABC Life's most successful series of all time. She was awarded the Arts Access Australia National Leadership Award in 2021.

Nina Tame

I was at a petting farm with my two youngest kiddos, the first time I'd been out with them in my wheelchair. My six-year-old was off with his dad, watching the lambs being fed, and I was chatting away to my toddler, who was in his buggy next to me. We were approached by a person holding a cute little baby chick. I say we, but it was really just my toddler, as apparently in that moment I had become completely invisible. I watched as said person began to pass the cute little baby chick to my toddler, and I said loudly and clearly, 'Please don't give him that. He'll try to eat it.' I was glanced at, dismissed, then watched as my son held out his greedy little mits, took the chick then immediately went to put it in his mouth. Told you so, Sandra. The chick was hastily grabbed back, and the person scurried away. That was the first time I realised that people didn't expect me to be a mum.

I'm now forty-one years old, and I have four kids, ranging in age from preschooler through to a young adult. (Yes, I am tired.) I was born Disabled with a condition called spina bifida. I used mobility aids on and off throughout my teenage years then things settled down in my twenties, so I stopped using them.

During my third pregnancy, one of my legs got weaker, so I began to use a walking stick. Fast-forward a few more years to my fourth pregnancy, and an unfortunate accident with some slippery tights and a hardwood floor, followed by another unfortunate accident with some hair straighteners and a foot I can't feel meant I upgraded to crutches and then my gorgeous wheelchair by the time my youngest was eighteen months old.

Wouldn't it be great if that was my story, a simple recounting of the mobility aids I use to help me as a Disabled parent. Alas, I'm a Disabled girl living in an ableist world, so you know it's juicier than that.

Looking back to my first pregnancy in 2004, I didn't even identify as Disabled, and my SB was something I tried to keep as hidden as possible. My own internalised ableism was huge, and the excitement of being pregnant was overshadowed with a sense of BUT. But what if the baby has SB like you? But what if the baby makes your SB worse? But what if you can't cope? Now, look, I get it, we're obsessed with 'healthy'. It's what people say isn't it – 'I don't care whether I'm having a girl or a boy as long as it's healthy'. So, the relief that my first two pregnancies were indeed 'healthy' was palpable.

Well, like a eugenicist's worst nightmare, I eventually (third time lucky) did have a baby like me. A gorgeous, wonderful, beautiful baby with spina bifida. I remember the doctor telling my partner and me in hushed tones as I lay on the table, my massive belly still covered in jelly, 'Your baby has SB. We don't know how serious it is. It might not be able to walk. Blah, blah,

blah. Would you like a termination?' There it was – offered right off the bat. A termination of my very, very wanted baby, purely because he was like me. I remember we laughed awkwardly and said of course not, but I was still offered a termination at each appointment that followed, right up until he was born. Because a life like mine isn't worth living? What a load of bollocks. He's now eight, and he currently does walk, but even if he didn't, a non-walking life is no less of a life.

I've never felt guilty for giving my baby SB, because I don't see my SB as a negative thing. I see my SB as a neutral thing which has sometimes led to amazing things and sometimes it's led to some shitty things. Most of the time, it's neither positive nor negative, it's just a part of who I am.

Not all doctors are quite as neutral about it as I was, though. The first doctor I saw after the birth of my third child burst into my cubicle without a hello. He just barked at me, 'Did you not take folic acid?' Folic acid prevents spina bifida.

I had taken it, but the accusatory nature of this little angry weasel meant I still burst into tears over my plate of mediocre hospital dinner. Thank fuck for the amazing neurosurgeon we saw six months later, who explained about folic acid not preventing all cases – in fact, it doesn't affect our type of SB at all. Our type of SB isn't even hereditary. A medical mystery, we are. Still, I feel the judgement, I see the looks, especially when we were both rocking matching leg braces for a while. Oh, the horror that I bred. How awfully irresponsible of me.

The series of unfortunate events I mentioned earlier meant I spent most of my fourth pregnancy in bed. I managed to wobble into one midwife appointment on two crutches, though. 'What's wrong with you, love?' she asked. Not quite having the words to tell her that nothing was fucking wrong with me, I told her I had spina bifida. Her eyes lit up in delight as she asked if she could have a little peep at the lump on my back that comes with it. Dear reader, I felt a swell of humiliation, being treated like a sideshow freak, but I also felt the power dynamics in the room. I lifted my top and let her have a good gawp.

For our next appointment, she visited me at home. Her greedy eyes lit up even more when she saw my son had SB too, and she started to ask him about it. So, I firmly told her, 'He doesn't want to talk about that. He's playing.' One hundred points to Nina. I still wish I could have told her to fuck right off, though.

Those early days with my fourth baby were at times tricky, but that's because I wasn't using the right tools for the job. I was still using crutches because again ableism told me that a wheelchair was a total horror show, and using it was an end-of-the-line decision. Or I'd use the pram for very slow, wobbly steps knowing I couldn't pick him up and lift him out if he needed a cuddle. We got by, though. I provided the sitting-down, milky-booby cuddles, and my partner, Jase, provided the standing-up, rocking ones. Friends or family would help me take him out, and my eldest would help me carry him up and down the stairs. That first year was mainly spent cuddling on the sofa until we moved to a bungalow, and I finally realised that crutches really weren't offering me the ability to live my best life.

So, I got a wheelchair. Oh, I love my wheelchair. Suddenly I could carry my not-so-little baby around. I could enjoy days out without constantly worrying I was going to fall over. The nerve pain I'd had in my legs for years went away. I regained freedom I hadn't had in such a long time. But the price for that? My identity as a mum was erased and my ability to parent was now hindered, not by my no-worky legs but by all the bloody access and attitude barriers.

People in wheelchairs are not generally viewed as being parents. Look at the mainstream media for a start: films, telly programmes, adverts. Where are the wheelchair parents? I think it's hard for society to view Disabled people as being parents for so many reasons. Firstly we'd have to be having the sex to have the babies, and for some reason Disabled people are all seen as pure and good and totally sexless. In reality, some of us are proper little filthy minxes having all the amazing saucy sex. Just like non-disabled people.

Then there's this idea that someone in a wheelchair must be totally broken. If my legs don't work, then surely nothing works. Again, the reality is that, just like non-disabled people, some of us can biologically have kids and some of us can't and some of us make the very valid choice not to be parents at all. Then of course there's the idea that surely if we need extra care, we can't possibly give care?

If people can get past these outdated attitudes and realise I am indeed the Mama then I am inspirational by default. Proper cream-your-pants inspirational. Someone saw me taking my kids to school once and cheered in delight. 'You're doing so well!!' They even felt it bore repeating when they saw me again ten minutes later, but this time they yelled it across the road at me.

I'd slept two hours the night before, because my toddler still thought my boobs were an all-you-can-eat buffet, and so I'd let the kids help themselves to breakfast out of the snack drawer that morning. But yeah, sure, I'm inspiring. (Actually, wait. Maybe that is inspiring.)

If I'm not serving up my best inspirational crip show then I am a joke on wheels.

Once we were out in London with the kids, the gorgeous wide smooth pavement an absolute wet dream for a wheelchair user, but also steep. The kind of steep you push through because you know the way back is gonna be an absolute joy. So, there we were, my youngest on my lap, us coasting down the slope, wind blowing in our hair and giggles escaping from our mouths, having an absolutely lovely time, when some hoity-toity middle-aged women in a posho neckerchief saw us and yelled to her friend, 'Oooh, mind you don't get run over.' As they chuckled to themselves, the urge to indeed run them over was strong. I resisted and we coasted past, but I was delighted when I heard Jase behind us loudly and sarcastically say, 'Oh, ha, ha, ha,' as he walked past them.

Then of course there are the access barriers, non-accessible playgrounds, schools and days out. Only being able to purchase one wheelchair space and a carer's ticket to a show (sorry kids, you'll have to sit on your own). Those diabolical platform lifts. I once took my then five-year-old to see a show at a venue where I'd experienced delicious access before. It was the first time we'd gone out with just the two of us, and I was thrilled to get to do this. Only, this time, there was a mix-up with our tickets. We were seated in the other disabled space, the one that required the use of a platform lift. I wheeled myself on, my little one was told to wait at the bottom of the stairs while a member of staff tried and failed to work the lift. Another member of staff was called, while the many other parents and their kids stared at the lady stuck at the top of the stairs and I reassured my kiddo that everything was okay. More staff came, the lift did not work and eventually we were taken to another one. That was the day I decided if I couldn't access something independently then it wasn't accessible at all.

Now let me tell you about the joy of being a Disabled parent, because there is so much joy. My youngest child's favourite game is riding around on my lap pretending Mummy is a bus. Or busting out some moves in our regular kitchen discos. You know kids' favourite things are wheels and bubbles, right? Some days our lives are beautifully slow and gentle, cuddles on the sofa with a good book, snuggling in a bed den watching cartoons or lazing in the garden doing some colouring. I mentioned the thrill of going down a hill, didn't I? My youngest is delighted when he sees another chair user, and he went through a stage of being really sad that he wasn't Disabled too. That was a strange conversation. 'It's okay, baby. You might be one day.'

I found myself chasing my two smaller kids round the house the other day in an epic game of 'Mummy is a scary giant', and one of my elder two remarked that we used to play that game when he was little. The only difference is now I'm playing it on wheels. This gives me the advantage of speed, although stairs are now my kryptonite.

The three eldest all know what ableism is, something that I didn't learn about until my mid-thirties. I love the mutual understanding and the smirks and eyerolls my teens give when someone says something predictably ridiculous to me. I love to hear how they talk to their friends about this stuff. They're not awkward around Disabled folks, they understand disability is a neutral thing, they don't automatically pity or feel inspired or any of the other nonsense that so many non-disabled people feel. I'm raising little allies and, honestly, it's the absolute best.

I do need extra help as a parent, especially during those early days. It's only now that my youngest is four and understands not to dart off into the road like the Flash that I feel comfortable taking him out on my own. It was hard, it IS hard some days to not get swept up in other people's highlight reels, to not feel a pang when I see a mother and kid doing something together that I couldn't do. I remember feeling a bit jealous once when my sister took one of the kids out for a day when I was going through a period of bed rest. I allowed myself to feel that hurt then reminded myself how lucky we were to have support to be able to do this. To put my pride to one side and remember that it takes a bloody village. No-one can be all the things, no-one can do all the things. We all have our strengths and weaknesses. I also remind myself that there's plenty of non-disabled people who get a ton of help with raising their kids, from childcare to live-in nannies, so if it's good enough for celebs then it's good enough for us Disabled folks.

Take away all the societal barriers, and my challenges as a parent who uses a wheelchair are the same as my challenges when I was a parent on two legs. I still stress that they mainly only eat beige breaded food. I worry I'm not giving them enough one-to-one time. I worry they'll grow up and make ridiculous choices and do a whole load of drugs just like I did back when I was wild and very silly. It's always a challenge to get them to do their homework, a challenge to peel them away from screens and a constant challenge to get the little one to stay in his own bed for a full night. (Secretly, I love him squeezing in with us. Being kicked in the ribs when I'm sound asleep? Not so much.)

Disability doesn't make you a lesser parent. That's just ableism whispering in your ear, and that guy's a total wanker. It's not a shame you're a Disabled parent, either. It's a shame we live in a hugely inaccessible world that totally erases Disabled parents. Disability weaves in and out of my parenting, the good and the bad. We make the needed adjustments; we lean on community for support and ideas. We find a way, and kitchen discos on wheels will always be the best.

* * *

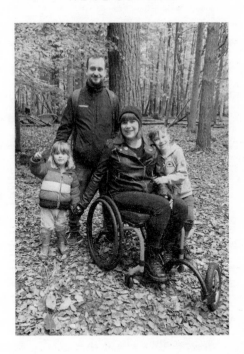

Nina Tame is a disability advocate, writer and content creator from the United Kingdom. She uses her Instagram account (@ nina_tame) to debunk outdated societal myths about disability and to explore the ways in which ableism features in her life. Her experience of growing up Disabled and parenting a Disabled child is a continual influence that runs through her work. With wit, passion and lots of wheelchair selfies, Nina's work explores the nuances of the Disabled experience while contributing to the growing, diverse and brilliant online Disabled community.

Sam Drummond

It takes me just six months to get to know my new neighbourhood. Not just the street names or where to get the best coffee, but each laneway, every shortcut, all the unmaintained bluestone paths. Which houses are home to hoarders, which businesses ignore 'no junk mail' signs and who mows their lawns on a Wednesday. This is the life of a parent whose child will only fall asleep in the pram. Come rain or slight drizzle, if I spot a yawn, a rub of the eyes or the pull of an ear, I whisk Young Me into the pram. Then the race is on – will she drift off to sleep or will my hips or knees give out first?

Watching her fall asleep is one of the great honours of parenthood so far. She stares at me intently with her indigo eyes. Her eyelids shut once, twice, then again for a final time – and she's asleep. That's on a good day. The alternative is that her eyes stay wide with wonder as we pass trees, dogs, birds. These endless walks inevitably result in another sleepless night. She will sleep like the proverbial baby she is. But my form of dwarfism means I will toss and turn from one sore hip to the other, trying to find the right angle for my swollen knee, stubbornly refusing painkillers because *I've had worse.*

Whether she falls asleep in the pram or not, there's always one thing at the back of my mind – I have a 50 per cent chance of passing this disability of mine on to her.

*

Being a parent was never really on the cards.

I hear this so often from other parents with a disability. Whether a disability is genetic, acquired or both, every disabled person gets subtle and not-so-subtle hints that they should not procreate.

The message that I am somehow 'lesser' because of my disability has been pounded into me for as long as I can remember.

In kindergarten, like in every kinder around the country, the teacher marked our heights against the wall, then ranked them from top to bottom. I was always last.

In the Grade 1 playground, another student told me their parents had warned them not to go near me because they might 'catch' my shortness. Anyone who has a physical difference knows that comments from young kids can be blunt and are not unusual. As an adult, I welcome questions and comments from children as an opportunity to make a positive impression. This particular interaction might have been one of a dozen schoolyard conversations about my appearance that week. It would not have stuck with me if it had not shown that adults – their parents – had the ignorance to hold such a view and then the bigotry to pass it on to their information-absorbing child.

Despite a love of sport, I was often sidelined from high school PE, plonked next to my classmate Kevin. Kevin's blood didn't clot, which explains why he couldn't participate in contact sport. It doesn't explain why no non-contact alternatives were offered. Other students were asked to push their physical limits while our limitations were fixed, defined by others. Kevin and I got the message that our own bodies were not something that fit in a teaching plan. They were certainly not something to be proud of.

Kevin died one school holidays in Year 8. Three of his classmates went to his funeral. I am ashamed to say I was not one of them.

And when it comes to sex, dating and reproduction for people with dwarfism, the message is not just that tall is better, but that it is tall or nothing.

Growing up, there was not a single media representation of a person like me as a healthy sexual being. Short-statured people, and disabled people more generally, have been forced to straddle competing stereotypes: either desexualised or fetishised. At one end, the child-like non-sexuality of the Oompa Loompas, the Seven Dwarfs or the *Wizard of Oz*'s Munchkins; at the other, hyper-sexualised Mini-Me from *Austin Powers*.

There is no doubt in my mind that these representations are at least in part responsible for the kind of life-shaping interactions that pulverise your confidence more than any schoolyard taunt. Like the drunk man at a music festival urinating on you 'because you're at the right height'. Or a crush telling you that you should be with 'your own kind' instead of her.

Through the way in which we are portrayed, the messages society sends to a young person with a disability is clear: you are different, you should be sidelined. If you are to succeed, it's not going to be with the rest of us.

If the messages don't get through to you by the time you're considering having kids, the 'genetic counselling' offered by health practitioners will do the trick. Even the name is a giveaway: you go to a counsellor when you have a problem (say, drinking), not when everything is hunky dory.

For reasons I cannot explain, my partner expressed so much interest in me early in our relationship, she wanted to accompany me to my regular specialist medical check-up. The doctor confirmed the maths to both of us without us even asking – if we had children, there would be a one in two chance that he would have a new patient. At that point in our lives, neither of us were interested in children. So it was to my relief that my partner smiled politely and declined an offer of genetic counselling.

I left that appointment knowing that the two of us had something special. Here was someone who was genuinely interested in everything about me. This interest was not just in the parts of my life that I enjoyed but also the ones I resented – like these inane medical appointments.

We were happy simply discovering each other. Sitting together with a cup of tea, a pack of cards and a warm blanket. I was the luckiest person in the world and didn't want anything to change. I certainly didn't want to do something as drastic as mention the possibility of children. That would be like being dealt a jack and an ace in blackjack, then saying to the dealer 'hit me'.

Being a parent was never really on the cards.

Until it was.

We had been on the trip of a lifetime, indulging every one of our senses in Malaysia, seeing orangutans and turtles in Sumatra, getting up close to elephants and blue whales in Sri Lanka, lazing on pristine beaches in Cambodia and even meeting the Sultan of Brunei on his Sunday morning bike ride. But it was a chance walk to a lighthouse in Penang that made me re-evaluate my priorities.

The local tourism website described the walk thus:

> The pathway up the hill from Monkey Beach starts off steep, but is nice and wide with steps, before narrowing into just a small narrow jungle track as you near the top. This is not a difficult trek and should take you 30 minutes to an hour depending on your level of fitness.

For me, fitness was not an issue. I had recently swum a marathon and had never been fitter. But while the tropical heat soaked us with sweat on the ascent, every step down from 227 metres above sea level to the beach jolted through my right knee like a spade hitting concrete. As my leg began to shake, my partner and I would embrace on each step and place our foreheads together, the way elephants do to show their love. She would then support my weight and lower me down to the next step. By the time we got to the bottom, after many more hours than the website had estimated, the damage had been done.

The pain I endured in the months that followed shaped our

trip. It would have been unbearable for my partner to watch. I had agency – I could focus on the pain and trick my brain into thinking these signals were harmless messages being sent from my leg. All my partner could do was be there with me and offer painkillers.

Each day, we would wake in a foreign bed and promise each other to take it easy. Then inevitably I would insist on walking through thick jungle or over the next hill, knowing all too well that this stubborn determination would end in agony.

People with disabilities and chronic illness know this sort of pain well. It makes you re-evaluate basic principles. And if you get out the end of it, you never approach life the same way again.

When I told people it made me realise my own mortality, I was often met with blank stares that said 'you didn't realise that already?' But this realisation was more than the obvious – it was the difference between a vague awareness that one day you are going to die and the complete acceptance of that fact. For me, this acceptance brought with it a sense of peace with the world around me and an urgency to make the most of the time I had left.

I arrived back in Australia with crutches and a renewed sense of purpose – the cards I had been dealt had changed and it was time to take a risk.

I decided that I should initiate 'The Talk'.

It turned out that we both thought the other didn't want kids. Each of us had been silent in the face of unquestioned assumptions. What about the teasing? The discrimination at school and work? The surgeries? The unending pain? How would I go lifting a child into a car seat or onto a change table?

What if they were able-bodied and could outrun me?

We cried.

We realised all these questions had been bogged down in the underlying assumptions placed on us by society.

The activist Stella Young, who we were both fortunate to be able to call a friend, had tattooed on her arm: *you get proud by practicing.*

Over dinners, trips away and midnight debriefs, my partner and I had regularly discussed the benefits that disability offers to our world. Our society falls into the trap of thinking the problem lies with the person with a disability when all the while the problem is a society that fails to fully accept and make adjustments for people with disabilities.

We live in a world that values sympathy for people with disabilities and encourages us to donate to hospitals so they can cure disability. Meanwhile, people with disabilities are left behind, because those things that would make life liveable – a translator, a piece of software, a ramp – are not given priority.

A world that embraces disability and empowers people with disability to live life as they choose is a world that is closer to seeing all of us reach our potential.

By focusing on these questions about whether society would accept another person with a disability, we were not practising disability pride.

We were accepting the view of an ableist world that sees disability as a burden.

We were denying the beauty that diversity of experiences brings our society.

For me, the decision to have a child was not in spite of disability. In no small part, it was *because* of it.

*

The journey of parenthood started by finding out that we were pregnant on the morning of a family funeral – a secret reminder between the two of us of the fragile cycle of life. It involved an ultrasound in which the radiographer, on learning about our kid's flip-of-a-coin chance of inheriting my disability, turned to my partner and uttered the words 'I'm sorry'.

My partner knows more than anyone that my disability makes me who I am and would not change a thing, so she replied: 'Don't be sorry, we've actually thought about this – we don't think it's a bad thing!'

*

Our daughter arrived in a world brimming with possibility. When I saw her squidgy face, I saw a person who could achieve anything, go anywhere, be anyone. Perhaps the process of ageing is simply realising the limits of what you can achieve, where you can go and who you can be.

The day she arrived, I experienced the full range of emotions that parenthood brings: absolute joy, exhaustion, pride, worry, protectiveness, love, and an emotion for which I do not know the word but which involves looking at your offspring and seeing yourself look back.

And then there was grief.

This last one is not something that is often spoken about, but there is so much to grieve – most notably the loss of your old life and the loss of future possibilities. I had expected this. It was a healthy part of letting go.

In her first breath my daughter caught whiffs of the bushfire smoke that had drifted from not too far east of us in Victoria. It circled the globe and spread back into every corner of our home from the west. In her first week, I grieved for the loss of being able to rely on a safe climate.

But there was also an unexpected kind of grief central to my disability. You see, our parenthood journey has involved a state of purgatory. If Young Me has inherited my disability, she won't start showing clear signs of it until she's about eighteen months old.

I was born within what the medical profession call 'the normal range of height', as was my daughter. This knowledge has brought with it a state of limbo in which I have grieved the possibilities that will be lost either way if she is able-bodied or if she is disabled.

If she does not have a disability, I have grieved for the part of her life that will miss out on the wonderful perspective and experiences that disability can bring.

If she does have a disability, I have grieved for the part of her life that will be defined by society's prejudice and expectations.

This is the dual burden of a genetic disability.

Either way, I have learnt that there is grief in parenting a child with a disability.

Those words jump out at me like a snake startled by a

bushwalker. My pre-parenthood self would hate this admission. I've listened to non-disabled parents talk about the sadness they felt when their child was diagnosed with a disability and dismissed them as arrogant or selfish.

But as I walk these endless backstreets, trying to get Young Me to sleep, I acknowledge that this grief is real. And as my knee buckles from the walking, I find that it's not just the prejudice she will face if she has a disability that causes me grief, but also the physical pain that potentially awaits her.

This is my moment of great doubt – can I have this grief and still be disability proud? It is all I can think about as I push the pram into the driveway, pick her up and walk straight to her room.

'I've had enough,' I call out to my partner, who is working from home in the next room. 'Something has to give.'

I put Young Me into the cot, look her straight in the eye and explain that we are about to learn a new way to go to sleep during the day. She cries. And cries. And cries. I pick her up and close my eyes, bowing my head towards hers. She quietens. To my surprise, I feel her forehead against mine, just like elephants do to show their love.

And then it clicks.

Before having a child, I thought that this journey was the ultimate act of disability pride. I was right, but for the wrong reasons. I didn't achieve pride just by having a child. Pride is something I have learnt through the love of this incredible being. She is completely present. She does not judge. She looks into my eyes and shows absolute devotion. She has reinforced the idea that you cannot love others without loving yourself too.

At one year old, she has inherited just about everything – my hair, my eyes, my love of books, my habit of continuing to eat as long as food keeps appearing on my plate. We still do not have confirmation of whether she has inherited my disability. But if it comes, it will not change a thing between us.

We will press our foreheads together like elephants and everything will be okay.

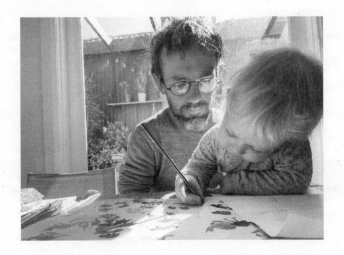

Sam Drummond is a lawyer and disability advocate. He lives in Melbourne with his partner Jo, daughter Gwendoline and dog Bessie. Sam and Gwen can often be found walking along Merri Creek, swimming at the Brunswick Baths or making friends with the elephants at Melbourne Zoo.

Micheline Lee

You are eight years old now, and for as long as you can remember I have been telling you the story of how we became your parents. In fact, I started telling you the story when you were still a baby, before you could even talk or understand, because I never wanted your adoption to come as a surprise or a revelation. I hoped the story would feel familiar and easy, like something you had always known. Not that I could have hidden it from you anyway, what with your big blue eyes and pale skin, and me with my Malaysian moonface. When you could talk, you would ask to hear over and over again stories about princesses and dragons, Aboriginal Dreamtime, Chinese emperors, giant bums and explosive farts. Sometimes, too, you would say, *now tell me about when you first saw me.*

I would start by telling you how the woman from the department rang me at work. *You have been selected to be the parents of a four-and-a-half-month-old baby!* she said. I couldn't believe my ears. She said we could meet you that very day at Pat, your foster mother's place. She gave me the address. You were staying just opposite our shopping centre in a house we always passed to get to the shops! It felt like I was dreaming. To think that I may have seen you already, sitting in a pram as I went by, and thought in passing *what a beautiful baby*, not knowing who you were, not knowing you would be ours. When I got off the phone I was crying tears of joy. Soon half my workmates were crowded in my office, hugging, jumping and laughing.

When your dad and I got to Pat's place, this is what we saw. You were lying in a bassinet, all plump, and in that dim light so pale your skin gave off a bluish tinge. The blinds were shut to keep out the heat of the Darwin build-up. You didn't make a sound, but you were wide awake and calmly waving a foot in the air. Three little Aboriginal girls surrounded you, the youngest still in nappies. The oldest girl, who looked about five, had her hand on your head. *He's my baby,* she said jutting out her chin and frowning at us.

Pat picked you up and handed you to your Dad. He was all long, pointy arms trying to find a way to hold you. At first you were still and silent, but soon you turned pink, then red, then purplish, and you opened your mouth wide into an almighty cry. Your dad handed you back to Pat and you sank into her cushiony body.

We didn't know who your birth mother was at that time. All we knew was that she carried you in her tummy for nine months; she gave birth to you, and she helped choose the parents who would adopt you. *These few things alone*, I said, *showed she cared very much for you.*

How you feel when you see me first time? you would ask when you were about five years old. I would tease: *well, I thought who is this fei toot toot, wat soot soot, pab loot loot.* You knew by then this meant 'plump, pale and soft', and was what your Chinese relatives said in singsong while cooing over you. The truth was I was just overwhelmed. Like the sky had opened up and showered us with manna and gold, and life had changed forever. That night, after meeting you, we lay awake in bed thunderstruck and speechless. We had not expected to be selected and had not prepared a thing. I was shivering though it was a hot, humid night.

We were fiercely committed to you from the moment we saw you. It took some days or weeks being with you, though, before you got under my skin, before I was totally immersed in love with your compact body, your smell, your every expression, your being. The first few days it was all very serious business – making sure we were feeding, bathing, changing and sleeping you right. But then we heard you laugh! Of all things, it was the sound of a plastic bag rustling near your ear that tickled your fancy. Your laugh sounded like the hee-haw of a little donkey. I liked to think you had finally relaxed. From then on, your delightful hee-haw laugh would erupt throughout the day for all kinds of reasons – grand, silly or mysterious – that somehow you found hilarious.

You especially could not stop laughing when you were swinging from the hoist in the air. Remember the pulley system I attached to the front of my wheelchair to pick you up off the floor? This was when you were crawling but couldn't stand or walk yet. I would hook you up to a sling, reel you up from the floor and swing you onto my lap. It took a month to design and build the hoist, and about two months for you to outgrow it. You learnt to crawl up to my wheelchair, climb onto the footrest, use the batteries under my seat as a foothold, and hurl yourself up into my arms.

Every time I told your adoption story, you had more questions. *Why my birth mother didn't want to keep me? Why Pat look after me? Am I Aboriginal like the sisters?* You started asking these questions by the time you were six. I'm not sure how much you could take in, but still I tried to answer your questions without glossing over all the hard issues involved in adoption and fostering. Again, I thought, even if you didn't understand everything, you would absorb it over time. The story grew to include more texture, more colour and more blurry lines. The funny thing was that although the story kept expanding, there were important parts I left out.

I never told you about how hard it was for me to apply for adoption. I never told you about how I may not have ever been able to adopt because people think that if you're disabled you can't raise a child. I didn't leave this part of the story out deliberately. Maybe it was just that I did not see the point in telling that part of it, because I had been immensely lucky to receive you and I was so grateful to be your mother.

People always look at us, curious about why we are together. *What is an Asian disabled woman doing with a Western boy?* they wonder. Most of the time, people are curious in an innocent or friendly way, but sometimes they treat us like we are suspicious or doing something bad. I am so used to it that most of the time I just ignore it. At first it didn't seem to be an issue for you, but about a year ago, when you began Grade 1, I started to notice a change. A few times when I dropped you at school or came into your class, I'd hear a kid say something to you like, *Who's she?* Or *What's wrong with her?* Or *She's not your mother!* At home you would be the same affectionate boy, but in school and in public you started to distance yourself from me.

Now, when I walk you to school and pick you up, I know that you don't want to be seen with me. I've never said anything about it to you, but of course I notice. You kiss me goodbye before we get to the bridge that leads to your school. *I can cross the bridge myself, you don't need to come with me*, you always say. But the school's rules are that I accompany you to the gate. I ask you to wait up, but you always race ahead over the bridge. When you were younger, we used to love lingering on top of that bridge, watching the cars whizzing by below, and looking down on the other side of the bridge at the kids playing in your schoolgrounds.

As soon as you reach the gate, you shoot away from me without a look over your shoulder. It's a similar deal when I come to pick you up. You just continue playing with your friends like you haven't seen me. But when I start coming towards you, you quickly say goodbye to your friends, pick up your bag and run out of the school gate as though you don't see me. Only when you get to the other side of the bridge do you wait for me to catch up to you.

Last week, when I fell out of my electric wheelchair at school, I don't think you saw what happened, but you definitely saw my wheelchair on its side and me lying in the grass. As usual, you were racing out the gate and I was following behind. You know the seatbelt that I put around you when I dink you on my lap? It came loose, got entangled in one wheel, pulled it to a halt and spun my chair around. I was thrown out of my chair. My knees slammed to the ground before I collapsed backwards. I couldn't move. Luckily, I fell on grass. So there I was, lying on my back with my legs twisted under me. I could see you on the top of the bridge looking down at me. Kids gathered. I asked them to get some adults to help me up. They came back with a teacher and a parent. They picked me up and put me back on my wheelchair. All this time you were up on the bridge, just standing there, watching.

On the other side of the bridge, I caught up with you. I was aching and shaken from the fall, and furious.

Why didn't you come to me when you saw me on the ground? I hissed.

You kept walking.

Stop and look at me when I am talking to you!

You stopped.

Why didn't you help your own mother?

Your poor face was contorted and you looked so lost. *I DON'T KNOW*, you shouted and ran away.

All I could think at the time was that you were ashamed of me. That you thought how pathetic I looked fallen on the ground and that you were embarrassed your friends and teachers had seen it too.

But I know now it was actually my own shame that was the problem. I didn't want you to see me like that, twisted and helpless on my back on the ground, needing to be helped up by the adults. I've tried so hard to be like the other parents. You know when it's my turn to come into class and cut the fruit for the kids to share? I'm the parent who turns up with the fruit already cut up and browning, because I don't want people to see that my arms are too weak to cut fruit.

When your dad and I applied to adopt a child, we feared we wouldn't have a chance. We had to apply for overseas adoption, because adoption of local children like you was rare. Every country had its own rules for who could adopt and who couldn't. Most of the countries said they would not accept people with disabilities as parents. And the countries that would accept applications from disabled people said they would only do so if their disabilities were mild.

We had to fill in what seemed like a million forms. The condition that causes my weak muscles is severe and degenerative. I deliberately didn't go to my usual specialist to fill out my medical form. I found a doctor with no specialisation in my condition who relied on my report of the symptoms of my condition and would agree that my disability was mild.

As part of the screening process, a social worker had to write a report on whether we would make suitable parents. He spent one day with us in our home, another session meeting extended family and another meeting our friends. I briefed everyone involved that we had to understate my disability and emphasise my independence to convince them my disability was only mild. I rehearsed and prepared for weeks in advance of the day that the social worker came to our home. He was going to have a meal with us. I was going to cook in front of him. Your dad and I arranged everything so it looked as seamless as possible. I chose to prepare a dish with vegetables that were tender enough I could cut them and I had rehearsed making their cutting look effortless.

Maybe I didn't have to try so hard. The social worker was completely relaxed, had his first gin and tonic at 11 am and kept going with three more until getting back into his car and leaving at 4 pm.

I'm not saying it's right to pretend you're something other than you are in order to be accepted. But the rules were unfair. It's discrimination to assume parents with disabilities can't raise children.

In the end, you, a Darwin child, became available, and we didn't have to be selected by a country overseas. We didn't expect to be selected as your parents. You see Western parents of Asian children, but it almost never happens that a Western child is adopted by an Asian parent. I am so grateful to those who selected us. I feel that maybe they understood how hard it would be for us to be selected through the overseas process and wanted to help us out.

I want to say how sorry I am that I got angry with you when I fell out of my wheelchair. How could I expect you to accept and feel comfortable with my disability when I couldn't do it myself! I was so scared of being seen as not good enough to be your mother. I shouldn't have got angry. I should have just explained that I could understand why you didn't come and help me, but I was hurting and really would have appreciated your help. Everyone falls and needs to be picked up sometimes.

I didn't apologise that day because it took some time for me to realise what was going on. We played cars on your bed together that night. You lined up your beloved Matchbox cars, arranged them in circles and zoomed them up and away. When you got tired, you held a little car in each hand and rolled them back and forth, back and forth, until you fell asleep. You didn't want any stories that night. But next time you ask me for your adoption story, I will include the parts about how people think you can't raise a child if you have a disability, and how they don't know what they're talking about.

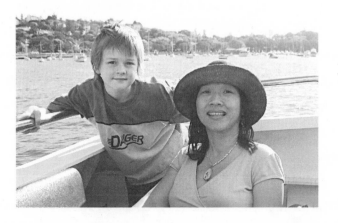

Micheline Lee's novel, *The Healing Party*, was shortlisted for the Victorian Premier's Literary Award; longlisted for the Voss prize; and shortlisted for the Dobbie Literary Award. Her essays have been published in *The Monthly* and in *The Best Australian Essays 2017*. Micheline migrated from Malaysia to Australia as a child. She has worked as a human rights lawyer and as a painter, before taking up writing. After fifteen years in Darwin, she now lives in Melbourne. Her son just turned twenty-one and still loves cars.

Lucy and James Catchpole

Our daughters are three and seven now – we're deep in the glorious, exhausting chaos of family life. This piece, though, is about becoming parents, how we were seen before as a disabled couple and how that changed with parenthood.

JAMES

Lucy and I were matchmade by a friend who has always said – only *slightly* defensively – that the match occurred to her *not* because we were both disabled, but because we had *other* things in common, and anyway she just thought we'd get on, alright? And our friend *was* right: Lucy and I have been married for fifteen years and counting. Not all of them have been plain sailing, but then life with disabilities often isn't. Having a similar starting point – being able to understand where each other is coming from – has been so important, especially when trying to navigate the storms.

On our first evening together, we worked out we had a lot in common . . .

- family background: gently, downwardly mobile;
- politics: somewhere between New Labour and raging Marxism;
- religion: lapsed Church of England vs lapsed Catholic (close enough);
- education: same university, though my schooling was a lot more expensive;
- books: she'd read them, and I'd at least heard of . . . most of them.

But when it came to our disabilities, we discovered our experiences could not have been more different.

I'm an amputee – missing all of one leg – and have been for as long as I can remember. I get around on crutches and am – well, was, at the time we met – fit and strong. I used to run on my sticks right across Oxford from my college to the university sports centre, where I kept a leg in a locker, and play badminton for two hours before locking up the leg and running back again. (The very idea now makes me wilt!) When I met Lucy, I looked dramatically different from the norm but felt as invincible as any twenty-three-year-old with no memory of ill health.

Lucy seemed to me, and I suspect to most people in her circle (and yes, she had a circle), like an infinitely sophisticated and capable twenty-four-year-old who appeared to know everything about the real world, could handle anything it threw at her and did it all while looking like Helen of Troy smoking roll-ups. She was also severely disabled by constant pain, was losing the use of one of her legs and was so physically vulnerable that a stray knock to the knee could permanently impair her mobility. She'd had a minor accident during a drama rehearsal in her second term at university, and her life had changed course overnight. But damn, she looked good.

She was consciously disabled. I'd grown up rejecting the label. She could pass as non-disabled, but needed a great many accommodations from society, for which she had to fight and fight. I looked properly disabled – no doubting my credentials – but needed nothing, and had to work hard to persuade old ladies *not* to offer me their seats on the bus.

Perhaps it's like Protestants and Catholics marrying: they're both Christian, but it's still a mixed marriage. We're both disabled, but ours has always been a mixed marriage too – certainly in terms of public perception. Well, that's not *quite* true. When I strap on my awkward, cumbersome robot leg to push Lucy's wheelchair, then we likely present as survivors from the same horrendous car crash. But as individuals, I've always been the supercrip, and she's always been the . . . well . . .

Lucy, what's the opposite of a supercrip? I'll leave her to answer that one!

For me as an amputee man, I've always found public perception to be ostensibly positive. You're thought of as heroic – superheroic, even. (Amputee Man – sounds like Marvel gone woke.) As a kid, you're 'amazing', 'a trooper'. In your twenties, people start assuming you actually *were* a soldier (especially if there's a war on, as there was during mine) and that you gave your limb for Queen and country. Then if you walk fast, climb stairs easily or do any kind of sport, you're 'inspirational'. And I don't only mean that in a shallow, Facebook-meme kind of way. Sometimes people seem to have profound experiences. The mere sight of you juggling a football can be an epiphany, apparently. And I know this because someone once wrote a letter to tell me so. I had been his burning bush, so to speak – which was good for him, if mildly confusing for me.

So that was my life as Amputee Man. But then I morphed into Amputee Dad . . .

As you might imagine, having a baby bobbing along, strapped to my chest, didn't exactly diminish this effect. It just added a new dimension. I think the difference is that between hero and saint. There's already a brilliantly unearned halo effect in being a dad out and about with a young baby. You're clearly doing better than just 'helping out', and that's enough to buy you some very indulgent looks. The bar is low, let's face it. Being a capable father of a newborn on one leg and crutches clears that bar with some room to spare. Forget writing letters: women have cried, then come over to tell me they are crying.

The flipside is when you drop the baby, of course. I haven't done this often – only once, and in fairness I caught her again. But enough people saw – and were horrified – to give me a pretty good idea that sainthood isn't necessarily a permanent state. I'd picked my moment well. A client of mine was speaking at the Oxford Literary Festival. I was there as supportive literary agent with baby obediently asleep in sling. So far, so saintly.

Then the baby woke up and pooped herself, and the poop leaked. Because of the crutches, I had to secure her in the sling to take her to the loo, and couldn't bear to strap her in too tightly, under the circumstances. I also had to cross the stage behind my client to get to the door. And of course, that's when she fell out – head-first. I caught her by the legs. A roomful of people inhaled audibly – a great, synchronised gasp. Bad dad. I caught the baby, but the halo crashed to the floor.

Lucy has had quite a different experience of public perception. People with her sort of disability don't often get to wear a halo like mine. There *is* one negative form of feedback that I've always had from strangers, though, which is perhaps worth thinking about in the context of parenthood. Missing a leg but looking otherwise 'normal' makes me into something of a walking question mark for a lot of people. They want to know what happened. They want a good story! I used to oblige, when I was young. Then I worked out I wasn't comfortable telling people, and that it wasn't any of their business. Eventually I even wrote a picture book about it.

Having kids in tow makes me inarguably a grown-up, and that discourages people from crossing lines, from forgetting their manners and indulging their curiosity. The fact that I'm far too busy trying to stop my kids from running down slides and playing in traffic helps too. Of course, this is counterbalanced by all the time I now spend in playgrounds, surrounded by other people's children, who are curiosity incarnate and couldn't care less how busy I am! Luckily I now have a handy shortcut for deflecting them: have you heard of this *excellent* book . . . ?

The thing about the question *what happened to you?* – even when asked in all innocence by a young child – is that it overturns the notion that people with bodies that look different from the norm might still have a normal expectation of privacy. And kids who don't learn this sometimes grow into adults who go much further: who march up to disabled people in public and ask them *can you still have sex?* Some disabled people get asked this a lot – women especially, I think. I've not had to deal with it often – one time in the post-office queue comes to mind – but having a high-level lower-limb amputation does seem to bring that question to the surface in people's heads. Back when the wars in Iraq and Afghanistan were going on and people used to ask me if I'd been a soldier, I suspect it was pretty easy to imagine I might have left more than just my leg by a dusty roadside in Helmand.

Happily, having your kids around does seem to put people's troubled minds to rest, on that score.

LUCY

I don't know what the opposite of a supercrip is, but whatever it is – I'm it.

James and I are both disabled, but our disabilities are very, very different – in the ways we experience them, yes, but what interests me more is the way we are perceived by the world around us. None of us is an island, we're all informed by the feedback we get from others – to an extent that constantly surprises me. And the world has always treated us very differently.

James is the epitome of the 'good disabled', as far as the world is concerned. When we met, James was a young, handsome Oxford postgraduate with one very clear whole leg missing. He used crutches with . . . elegance, strength. He needed no accommodations. You simply had to adjust slightly to the unusual shape of him, and that was it. And honestly, that asymmetry was visually rather pleasing, if you ask me.

And isn't that just the dream disabled person, really? A whole leg missing – the clarity of it!

But like many disabled people, I have always been a category error. Where James looks splendidly, unapologetically disabled, when we met I could pass as non-disabled but actually was very, very limited. The bad disabled. The hard-to-categorise. With pain – a lot of pain.

People seem to find significant disability that is also invisible particularly challenging.

Since we met, my disability has changed. I'm now a full-time wheelchair user – still difficult, with my pain and my need to exist horizontally most of the time, but if I'm seen as a burden, I'm at least a legitimate burden(!). An explicable one.

As a couple out in public, we've always been very visible. But the way we've been seen has changed along with my level of disability. We've lived a few different phases now.

At first I appeared to be the non-disabled girlfriend of an amputee. Before we met, I'd had to plot and wheedle my way to a desperately needed seat. Now, with a one-legged man next to me, people sprang out of chairs the moment they saw us. I remember one man vaulting over a table in his eagerness to give us a seat in a pub. The presumption was that I was the 'carer'. (God knows what they thought when James then gave *me* the chair.)

Then we were both crutch or walking-stick users. People

wanted to know how we met: 'Oh, you mean at some sort of special club or something?'

After that, the tragic phase: a wheelchair user pushed by a man with an artificial leg. Had we been in some terrible accident? Were we out on day release from somewhere or other? Happily, most people were too polite, or awkward, to ask.

When people did intervene, it tended to be more . . . physical. There is no taboo about grabbing disabled people: moving us without our consent – as though we're trolleys, or suitcases. So we had to work hard to stop well-intentioned people attempting to 'help'. (Game face on – fixed smile, signal absolute confidence. Say 'NO' cheerfully but emphatically at every approach. With warmth in your voice, because nobody likes a grumpy cripple.)

This final pre-children phase was unifying. Out in public, we dodged the wheelchair grabbers together. But the reality the rest of the time was the same as always: James on his crutches, still a supercrip, and me, still . . . the opposite.

However far removed these perceptions are from reality, from who each of you are as individuals and from who you are together, they still chip away at you. As I moved from suspiciously questionable disabled person to full-time wheelchair user, James's status as supercrip could only be further cemented. I know he found this awkward and tried not to let it affect how he saw himself. ('Yup, I'm basically a saint,' he once said sarcastically to a visitor whose praise-of-James speech had gone on quite long enough.) But it couldn't help having an impact. And likewise, the very clear message I got, from just about everywhere, was that I was difficult and burdensome. And lucky, very, very lucky, to have James. (I mean, I don't disagree, but it's not exactly tactful.)

Parenthood was something I desperately wanted. We both did. And feared it too. For both of us, putting my capricious, fragile body through pregnancy and birth was terrifying.

But for me, there was an extra dose of fear. I was completely used to my position as the weak partner, the 'difficult' one, in the world's eyes. And let's face it, with expectations of fathers already so low that parenting your own children is applauded, James becoming a father was hardly going to redress that. So, honestly, I was terrified of the world's response to my pregnancy. And to my motherhood, which would never be of the complete, twenty-four-hour-a-day variety. I couldn't imagine any response to pregnant-me, or to mother-me, that didn't pile on more confusion and disapproval.

If becoming a nice straightforward full-time wheelchair user had somehow redeemed me in the eyes of the world by giving me a clearly defined category, I could see no way that pregnancy wouldn't send me right back into the other, 'difficult disabled' one. Really, the idea that I would selfishly use my difficult, burdensome body to grow an entirely new human – completely unnecessarily – felt like taking the piss.

And we both knew I wouldn't have the stamina to be the primary parent. I could not have been more aware how far outside the norm that was. I expected to be condemned for burdening James further, and for creating children I couldn't parent on my own. (*Oh, that nice young man with one leg – what a shame he couldn't have found some nice strapping lass instead.*

Someone who can carry babies and bound upstairs. That sort of thing.)

When I was pregnant, I steeled myself for our first, difficult meetings with midwives and doctors. (Smile, perform femininity, perform brave disabled person, speak – but not too much.) I expected to have to justify my decision. I expected them to divide and conquer – sympathetic glances towards James and 'but how are YOU?'. I expected all of this because we'd been here before. This was just what happened in my medical appointments. I was a problem, I was infantilised. James was . . . well thank goodness for James! (That last bit is a quote. I heard it a lot.)

But that isn't how it turned out.

When we went for my first scan, instead of the disapproval I expected, the doctor scanning me responded very, very differently. 'I don't think anyone could fail to be impressed by you,' he said. Not to James, to us. To ME. This was very, very new.

Somehow, by becoming pregnant, I had jumped out of the difficult-disabled category and joined my husband in the supercrip camp.

And perhaps more importantly, we were now being seen as a unit. An 'impressive' unit. Together. As a couple, we were finally a fait accompli.

Life rarely changes all at once, and I don't want to oversimplify. This was not an immediate shift. When our daughter was a baby, I caught intense looks of concern and confusion, the occasional half-lunge when someone really, really wanted to take this precious newborn away from the lady in the wheelchair.

But once our first child was tottering around and saying 'Mama', I felt any disquiet from the world calm.

I did not expect motherhood to legitimise me. And yet it has. I think motherhood, or at least my motherhood – as the wheelchair-using mother of non-disabled children – acts to cancel out a lot of the things about me that the world found so disquieting.

There are so many ways disabled people are infantilised – we're frequently just not seen as adults. But now, where I had been infantilised, my children seemed to act as an automatic pass to adulthood. Legitimacy.

It felt like a magic time to me, when our babies were still babies and could ride on my lap. I momentarily encompassed the same contradictions that make James so appealing to people. My evidently 'broken' body had created a life, just as James's 'incomplete' body was nonetheless agile and strong. A strange, magical time. My temporary passport to supercrip status.

I thought this would disappear once the clear through-line from me to pregnancy had gone – once the baby was no longer a baby. But now when we go out, the children are like unselfconscious ambassadors, skipping along with us, signalling my normality to the world.

We are still very visible. Probably more so, with the whole roadshow of now: two adults, one working leg between them, and two children. More children than working legs, in fact. But where I expected motherhood to open me up to even more judgement, it has had the opposite effect. Where people once thought they saw a vulnerable couple to be pitied . . . well, I don't know quite what they see now. But we're manifestly parents. We've evidently grown and kept alive these darting, energetic creatures – our daughters.

It troubles me sometimes. I am unchanged. I still live, mostly, in bed. My pain levels are just as high, I am just as susceptible to injury, my – rational – fear of anyone inadvertently hurting me is just as great. But whereas before, these elements of my life were treated with awkwardness, as though they were an eccentricity, to my great surprise now I am taken seriously.

Society's feelings about women and motherhood and birth and pain are pretty unreconstructed, really. Is it, I wonder, only now that I've gone through pregnancy and birth, that my perception of pain is accepted as . . . valid? And so if I say something hurts, it probably does? I don't know how else to account for the difference in tone in my interactions – with medics, especially.

And how is it that I am seen now as less of a burden on my husband than before, when I still have to rest for much of the day, and he does most of the nappy-changing and feeding? Perhaps I still would have been seen that way if James had looked careworn instead of springing into fatherhood, glowing with the joy of it. But I think I also missed something about the status mothers have. No, compared to fathers, mothers are not given an easy time of it. But society also respects motherhood. It can act as a powerful talisman, being a mother, or as protective armour, trumping other parts of your identity.

It is irrational, that the world should view me so much more kindly, with so much more respect, just because I've now had children. But it is also irrational that people cry at James in the street. And that I was viewed with such suspicion as a disabled person, until I became unable to walk.

There's very little any of us can do to change the judgements people make about us. And we can't deny they affect us – how could they not? These are the constraints we all live within. They're dictated by a whole host of things – race, class, the way we look, the nature of our disabilities – very little of which we can control. Choosing to have children throws all of that up in the air, reconfiguring it. We've been lucky that the world around us responded the way it did – there was no guarantee.

It was a risk, becoming parents – it is for anyone, of course, but there are many more unknowns with disability in the mix. The cliches are true, and it's hard to write about parenthood without slipping into them – it *is* a leap into the unknown, it *does* change everything, it *is* a relentless, gorgeous bombardment of joy and exhaustion and chaos and love. But even with a surprise global pandemic and two years of unexpected homeschooling, it's still the best shared project we could have imagined. And in our experience, if you can weather disability together, you're probably well equipped to weather parenthood.

I am so very, very glad we took the risk.

* * *

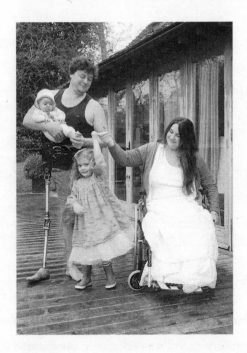

Lucy and James Catchpole live in Oxford, England, with their two daughters, and run The Catchpole Agency for authors and illustrators of children's books. Lucy has written about disability for the BBC and *The Guardian*, and James is the author of the picture book *What Happened to You?* They have co-authored a sequel, *You're So Amazing*. You can find them @thecatchpoles on Instagram.

Cathy Reay

from an interview with Eliza Hull

I have an older brother and sister from my dad's previous marriage, but we weren't raised in the same home. I saw them every other weekend when we were young, but that petered out as they grew older and got busy social lives. So I've always viewed my childhood a bit like that of an only child, and that was both a privilege and a weight.

I'm lucky to have very loving parents. They're non-disabled, but they have always accepted me for who I was, disability included, which I know isn't always the case in our community. Yet I still felt very imprisoned by our small nuclear-family structure, especially during my teens.

I grew up in a very poor rural area of eastern England, where families tended to be large, and familial relationships are very important. I wanted that sense of community that my peers had. I wanted siblings to bicker with; others my age I wouldn't have to be nice to because they were blood relatives. I wanted to share my things. I just wanted to experience that joy of a bustling, noisy home.

As I grew older, I moved on to desiring my own children who would create that bustling, noisy home I had always craved. But I was conflicted by the ableism I faced, both in society and internally.

For a long time, I believed I would never have the chance of falling in love or getting married. I knew I could have children, because I knew other people with dwarfism who had them, but after a string of failed relationships and complete nonstarters, I didn't think I would ever meet somebody that would want to have children with me.

When I did eventually fall in love, our relationship blossomed sure and fast, as did our family. It was like I'd been holding my breath and I could suddenly exhale. My dreams were finally coming true.

People with achondroplasia, which is the type of dwarfism I have, have children by caesarean section. My partner and I both worried about how I would recover, how I would manage the physical part of being a parent, such as holding the baby, lifting them up when they got a bit older and ensuring they kept out of danger. He was concerned about my physical ability to take care of our kids, even though I'd already done so much in my life to date completely independently. But to be honest, these things were a worry for me too. I know that I'm incredibly resourceful and resilient, and my body has been through loads, but I'm also aware that there are things that are naturally, undeniably harder. And I think when you're presented with parenthood so suddenly – because there's no other way to be presented with it – the unknowns of what might be hard are scary. These worries were never a reason to deter either of us, though. We were excited, but also apprehensive.

My approach to life has always been very 'fools rush in'. I don't tend to research things, I just go for it and hope for the best. I didn't read any pregnancy literature, I just went along with it.

For my first, there was a doctor at the local hospital that knew a bit more than the average GP about my disability. However, they weren't always on hand for all my appointments. I remember being at an ultrasound scan and my doctor's stand-in asked me, with a very serious look on their face, 'You know, it looks like the baby is going to have dwarfism, is this something that's going to be a problem for you?' I was taken aback. What they were really saying was, *This baby has something wrong with it – do you want to keep it?*

Because I have dwarfism myself, it stung. The fact that the question was even asked made me realise that society hasn't progressed that far. It was a reminder that people view our lives as faulty and less than. It was a reminder of how the medical system is not set up to support disabled children and their families. I felt so othered, and I worried that my baby was going to experience that too.

When I was seven months pregnant, I fell over on the way to work, landing on my stomach. As soon as I stood up, I had a horrible feeling that something wasn't right. I wanted to check everything was okay, so an ambulance was called. The paramedics called through to the hospital, but staff there refused to see me. I had to really fight to be taken seriously, and eventually the hospital agreed to see me. When I got there, they did a scan, and found that the baby was suffocating, so they performed an emergency caesarean.

My maternity cover at work hadn't started yet. Nothing was ready in the house. Anyone that knows me will attest to the fact that I am a last-minute person. I felt incredibly overwhelmed, and ended up having quite severe postnatal depression after the birth, attributed largely to the sudden and very scary nature of that experience. I also didn't have any of the medical team that I had planned to have there.

My birthing experience felt very undignified and at times unsafe; it was one of those times where you're so severely reminded that you know your body better than anybody. Pushing for that, for what you need, is so important, but can be so exhausting.

When I was having the C-section, I remember telling the staff that I needed to wee, so they told me they would insert a catheter. I tried to tell them that it wasn't in properly, insistently telling them that I needed to wee and couldn't wait, all while they were pushing down directly onto my abdomen trying to get the baby out. They shushed me and said no, it's just the drugs telling you that, go ahead and wee, and then I urinated all over myself and them. Because they didn't listen to me, I had to lie in a pool of piss as my baby was delivered. That wasn't how I envisioned the birth, and after everything that I'd been through on that day, I felt sad and defeated. The doctors came to apologise to me afterwards, but the memory remains.

Luckily, when I had another child, I carried her almost to term and she was born by planned caesarean section. That birth was a lot easier. Because both my babies were born before full term, it meant that my body didn't carry them at their heaviest, so it was inevitably more manageable for my smaller body.

When my children were little, the physical toll their existence took on my body was unexpectedly hard. I was very naive about it. I thought it would be fine because I had such smooth pregnancies. But for the first three or so years of each of their lives, I was in an immense amount of pain. Especially when I had my second. I found that immeasurably hard on my body. I have never recovered from that. I've always been a tired person, even when I was a kid, but the lack of sleep, coupled with always needing to carry them, run with them, move with them – it absolutely drained me.

I think you can have an idea of how you'll be as a disabled parent; you might be able to prepare in some ways. But you don't really know until the time comes. A lot of things can be adapted or changed to fit around us, but some can't. I found it hard finding a buggy because most of them aren't low enough for me to see over. After searching, I eventually found one that was the right height, although there was a different problem: I couldn't lift the carry cot out of the buggy and fold it. I don't drive, so I never had to put it in a car, so I just never packed it down. Disabled people are the most resourceful I know; we're always finding ways to alter processes to make them accessible for us.

My first child had a drop-side cot, so when it was bedtime I'd just put down the side and put her in. This design was made illegal in the United Kingdom, so my second kid slept on a mattress on the floor. Everything was done on the floor for the first year, including nappy changing. It was so much safer, although it was a killer for my back because I was bending over all the time.

I think one of the biggest ways I adapted was to slow down. And rest more, which I'm historically not very good at. I'm definitely somebody who overworks and defines their self-worth by their work a lot of the time. And I just couldn't when they were super young.

Becoming a single parent was another readjustment; everything we had done together now had to be done alone. I was very fortunate to be in a position to pay for somebody to look after the kids when I was working or needed to go out. This has been invaluable for me physically, as well as mentally and emotionally, because it gives my body a chance to rest. Even when I'm working, it affords me that chance to recuperate. As a solo parent, weekends can be hard for me; by Sunday night, my entire body aches.

My kids are now eight and four years old. They know that I am proudly disabled. I don't identify as disabled, I am disabled. I feel quite strongly about that terminology. Because identify kind of implies to me that you can switch it on and off. That's not my experience. I've always been disabled. I haven't always had the language that I have now, but I've always had the beliefs that I have, and that's largely due to my parents raising me to understand that 99.9 per cent of barriers I face as a disabled person have nothing to do with my body. They taught me that society was the issue.

My daughters knew early on that we are all disabled. I've always named our disability, and we talk through the things that can be frustrating for us in inaccessible environments, and the negative reactions we receive. Sometimes I find it hard grading my language with them and drawing on examples they fully understand. Ultimately, though, they get it, because it's their lived experience too.

Since they have started connecting with other children at school, non-disabled parents don't know what to do with me, because I am defying all the things they think about disability. I am pushing up against misconceptions like 'disabled people don't have sex' or 'no-one would ever be attracted to a disabled person' or that 'disabled people can't conceive' and 'disabled people can't look after other people, they can't have dependents.'

I think because of these misconceptions people are a bit like, 'Whoa, what *are* you?' And they're afraid. People are scared of disability in general anyway. Everyone's afraid they might catch it, might be asked to do something for us, or might say the wrong thing. But they're really afraid when they see a disabled person living, doing stuff. By me just existing in society in my disabled family, people are like, 'Whoa, what is going on?'

This isn't how people actually talk to me; it's just what I imagine they're thinking, based on their very clear avoidance to interact with me as a parent in places such as the school playground. I think people don't know what to do. I also think there's an element of people thinking that they're going to make a mistake and mess up in the conversation, so they just don't talk to me because they're scared. Many people think people with dwarfism are infantile, because of our size, or freaks, because of our long-running association with pantomime. We are rarely thought of as sexy or lovable or even adult.

Being a single disabled parent probably makes sense to the more ableist people. Like, 'That makes sense – he got kids out of her then left.' This couldn't be further from the truth, but it's not my job to make people see that. If I was still in a romantic relationship with the father of my kids now, I would definitely not experience as much exclusion from other parents – women, particularly.

It can be hard being a single disabled mum. At times it's very lonely. Thanks to ableism and single-parent stigma, I don't really feel part of the motherhood crowds, and my disabled friends are too scattered to see often. Women in particular are fed this goal of finding a partner and settling down and having a family and having a good career. But if that family breaks up, that's when you realise how hard it is to do it alone. It's really challenging to juggle everything. But for me, the hardest thing has been the loneliness. Not having someone to bounce things off; someone who is equally invested in the day-to-day mundane stuff of parenthood, someone who is there with a glass of wine waiting for you after bedtime. While I don't necessarily want a cohabiting relationship in that way anymore, I can certainly see the value it brings when raising children together.

Being a disabled parent, I like to think that I bring resilience and resourcefulness and compassion and grace for myself and others. That's what I try to teach my children anyway. I think being disabled and having such a positive outlook on disability, sometimes a negative one, or a neutral one, models the true ups and downs of what it's like. It speaks volumes that they can see me living my life and achieving things that I want to do with the same disability that they have. And, that they see me, and they hear me talking about my views on disability in a radical way, and while they might not always understand or agree, my hope is that they will always be very rooted in what they believe, and unafraid to live that.

We have a lot of conversations about disability; we also have conversations about race and gender. My kids are marginalised in more ways than I am, and it's vital that I help them to understand their disability, their race, their gender. Their identity as a whole is never the problem – ableism, racism and sexism are.

They're both very aware that they're disabled. People's attitudes are something I constantly have to navigate with them as a parent. I talk to them often about the issues, about accessibility and ableism. Sometimes they have days where their attitude is more like: if someone's got a problem with me, it's their problem. Other times they internalise it a bit more. I've been trying to work on that with them, explaining to them that if people laugh at us in the street, it is their problem, not ours. Of course, it affects us sometimes, but longer term I try to instil an inner confidence in knowing who they are and not letting others dictate how they feel about their bodies. We all have days where we feel negatively about ourselves, and it's unrealistic not to expect that to happen. It's just important to remember overall that who we are is never the problem.

When kids are very young, especially kids with dwarfism

because we're so small, everyone coos and says, 'Aww, they're so cute.' As we mature and our faces lose that babyish charm, everyone's like, 'Oh, what's wrong with them?' There's a very definite shift for people like us. From cute babies to freaky adults.

I wanted to be a parent because I wanted brothers and sisters, I wanted a noisy house. I wanted to be a parent because society told me that's what I should do. I wanted to be a parent to have little people to love who would love me back.

While I absolutely don't regret having children, I wish I had understood more of what it was like. I know it's hard to understand without just . . . doing it. But I do wish I had sought out a bit more of the experiences, especially within my community, and properly talked to people about the realities of it. I don't think I necessarily would have made different decisions, but I think it would have been easier, especially for the first pregnancy and then the subsequent months after.

Having fun and being silly with my kids is the best thing about being their mum. The intimacy and freedom that comes with living in the moment, laughing uncontrollably about something together – it feels incredible. It's like we're laughing in the face of anything and anyone in our way.

Watching them unapologetically being themselves and knowing that I contributed to part of that light, and that they're going to be amazing adults, and they're going to do incredible things . . . nothing else beats that.

* * *

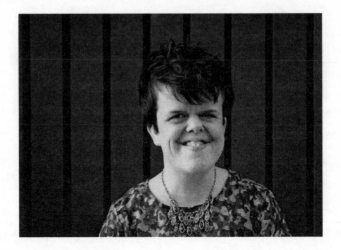

Cathy Reay is an editor and writer based near London. She began her writing career working for a disability journal and local newspapers, and then moved into online journalism and the national press. She is a queer, polyamorous single parent of two awesome humans.

Christa Couture

from an interview with Eliza Hull

When I was little, I wanted to be a mom. As a child, it's very easy to pretend-play getting married and having children because that's the stories we are told.

At eleven years old, I was diagnosed with Ewing's sarcoma, a rare form of bone cancer. I underwent chemotherapy and radiotherapy and went into remission, but then it came back. When I was thirteen, I had to have my leg amputated above the knee, which was the cure for my cancer but also an enormous loss. It felt like an exaggerated version of adolescence, in that I was already questioning 'What is this body? Who am I in the world?' And suddenly, I was someone with one leg. My whole life changed. My friends were having their first boyfriends, and I was just going to rehab hospital in order to learn how to walk again. I felt like I was set on a very different path than my peers.

My dad lived in New Jersey, so it was mostly just my mom and me. She was a single mom and had a child with cancer. Now I wonder how she managed. She did such a good job of keeping her fear and grief separate from me. I'm sure that she went through a grieving process and was scared and overwhelmed. It would have been a lot on her plate, but she was so supportive. I remember the day that I was going in for my amputation. It was all happening very fast: only four days after tests confirmed the cancer was back, I had to have the surgery. I got up in the morning, and Mom had written me a card that was on the counter. It said, *Today you're going to become cancer free. And from now on, you have a new body that's a healthy body.* It was the most beautiful, positive message. I think my mom really did the best she could. I didn't see her despair, I didn't see her go, *Oh well, you're screwed.*

By eighteen, I was in remission and had long-term follow-up care. I remember my oncologist at the time giving me this list of all the possible long-term side effects of the chemotherapies I'd had, and one of them was that it would be difficult for me to conceive. He said I shouldn't wait too long to begin trying, otherwise I would need interventions.

I spent my twenties thinking I wouldn't be able to get pregnant. And then I had an unplanned pregnancy, and I was like, *Wait a second. I've been careless, because I thought I can't get pregnant. But I can,* so that information was not a contraceptive. I terminated that first pregnancy, but it reintroduced the idea to me of having children.

In my late twenties, I fell in love. I remember we'd been dating only a couple of months, and we drove past these houses I really loved in my neighbourhood. I told my love that I thought it'd be cool to live there, and then I automatically said out loud,

'But I could never have kids there, because they have a lot of steps. I don't know how I'd get a stroller up and down those stairs.' Then I paused because we were so new, and said, 'I mean, if I have kids one day.' In that moment, he looked at me and said, 'I want to have kids one day,' and I replied, 'Me too.' It was a lovely moment in our early days of imagining a future together.

After that, I had a second unplanned pregnancy. We'd only been dating six months.

At first I struggled with the fact that I was pregnant. Even though I wanted the baby, I wasn't ready. I'm a singer and had just recorded my first album, I was planning on going on my first tour. I felt like everyone around me was starting to have their careers take off, and I was going to have a baby. But thank goodness it takes nine months; in that time, I got used to the idea.

As I got bigger and bigger, it became more difficult physically. No matter if you have a disability or not, pregnancy is a lot for the body. It was summer in Vancouver, and I was so pregnant, I was just melting in the heat being so uncomfortable and feeling so left out from what my friends were doing and grappling with it all.

After a complicated labour, our son Emmett died when he was just a day old. Suddenly all that stuff, that grappling, that struggling, didn't matter. I remember thinking, *Just because I was unsure doesn't mean I didn't want this baby.* His death shifted all that difficulty and all the emotional reckoning and the physical challenges. I wanted my baby. I wanted him and now he was gone. It put everything into perspective, it didn't matter that it was hot. It didn't matter that it was uncomfortable. Because losing him was so heartbreaking. All those pieces got all tangled up: the grief of not planning to put my career on hold, but now that I could go back to my career, I didn't really care.

I didn't know if I could risk losing a child again. I didn't know if I could be open to another loss. So much of pregnancy and childbirth is out of our control. But at the same time, since I had lost Emmett, I had this ache in me that desperately wanted to be a mother. Emmett illuminated this part in me that I didn't even know existed. *Oh, this is what it feels like. This is what love is.* And then with him gone, what had been illuminated now just ached. But my partner and I decided to do some things for ourselves, he wanted to do his MFA, and I was recording another album, so we decided to take some time.

But then we had another unplanned pregnancy.

The minute I knew I was pregnant the third time, I was just so ready and wanted it so badly. My son Ford was diagnosed in utero at five months with hypoplastic left heart syndrome. When he was just nine days old, he had open-heart surgery, then more surgery at four months old. It was incredibly challenging and scary. And it was incredibly joyful, too, to have him.

The first time we were able to take him home from the hospital, he was already six months old. But it only lasted a couple of weeks, and he was back in the hospital. His life was medically really challenging.

We knew that he would have several developmental delays, so we had things in place like physio and speech therapy. I was so ready to parent a disabled kid. Having him helped me feel more acceptance of my own disability because he was perfect. He was a perfect baby. And I loved him and wanted him to be safe. And it made me think about times that I'd resented or grappled with my own disability. But he had a difficult life, and a lot of things kept going wrong for him. He died when he was just fourteen months old. We just had really bad luck, to put it mildly. Devastating luck, really. A lot of my experience with motherhood has been so incredibly heartbreaking.

These losses were too much for me and my husband. Our lives fell apart, and our marriage ended. At the time, I was living in Vancouver and decided to move to Toronto to start over. I'd lost Emmett, I'd lost Ford, part of me wondered, *Will I ever be okay? Can I be okay and not have a child?* I started wondering, *Maybe there's other things I can have in my life. I can have a fulfilling beautiful life and not have a child. Or do I want to try for another child? Can I be open to another loss?* These are the questions I was asking myself, and I wasn't partnered. To consider trying to have another kid, I had to be able to be hopeful, I had to be able to believe it could work out. It took me a long time, but eventually I felt clear that I wanted to try, that I was open to whatever would come. I decided to become a single mother by choice.

I did an intra-uterine insemination (IUI) with anonymous donor sperm and got pregnant on the first try.

It was a high-risk pregnancy because of everything that had happened. But I was watched so closely and cared for so well, and the pregnancy was totally smooth. I remember my cousin saying at one point, 'Is this a good idea? You're disabled, you're single.' And I remember replying, 'It's going to be fine.'

When I was pregnant, I met a woman named Marsha and

we started dating. It was a bold, brave choice we made to start a relationship when I was about to have a baby, but Marsha was there when I gave birth to a beautiful little girl, Sona.

Marsha parented with me from the start, but over time we realised that we weren't going to be the best together as partners, although we decided to continue to co-parent. She adopted Sona as a step-parent and will forever be her other mom. I was ready to be the single disabled mom, I was going to make it work. But this queer family love story happened, and now this little kid has two parents. The more people who love you, the better. I feel incredibly lucky that our family formed this way.

I didn't really know until I had Sona how physically demanding parenting would be. Because Ford had been in the hospital the whole time, the demands weren't the same as parenting at home. I hadn't really let myself think about what it's like to get up and down off the floor constantly and carrying someone that just keeps getting bigger and heavier. Or even trying to go on long walks with a stroller because you just want them to fall asleep. I just couldn't really do all of that. Turns out, the physical demands were really difficult, and I was in a lot of physical pain the first couple of years trying to keep up. I would have done it all on my own, but I am so glad I didn't have to.

I remember Sona noticing I had only one leg when she was just under two. We were playing on the floor. She was standing on my lap, and I was holding her hands. First she stood on my right leg, then she stepped on the other side and stepped on my prosthesis, and then she looked up at me surprised because it felt so different under her feet. She continued moving her feet around my legs, discovering that they felt different, which I thought was really interesting, because she obviously hadn't thought that they looked different.

Now I talk about my stump and my prosthesis and my crutches and it's normalised for her. She has never asked what happened or why it's different from most other bodies she sees, though. I often wonder what will happen when she hears those questions. Usually they get asked by other kids or other people out in the world, and they're something I've become less tolerant of: I don't like when I'm in a playground with Sona and people come up to me and start asking about my leg and want to touch my prosthesis.

I'm excited to see how she describes it to other people one day. I love that it's normal for her, I hope that it stays that way. And I hope that that means other differences will be less surprising to her.

I try to talk to her about my limitations in the way that hopefully she can be compassionate about. If there's something we want to do, I will sometimes say to her that's not something I can do today, because this part of my leg is hurting me today, so let's do that tomorrow. I see her computing that information; she's increasingly understanding. Sometimes I'll ask for her help, and she'll help me, and I'll explain why I can't do a thing, I think it gives her perspective of how it's good to help people when they need it. I also hope my having a disability introduces her to the fact that all bodies are different, that it normalises all bodies for her.

Because I can't do the big physical things with her, and there are times that I can't get up and go places with her, I've become expert at creating a world sitting in one spot. A world for just the two of us, right here. Our beautiful world.

* * *

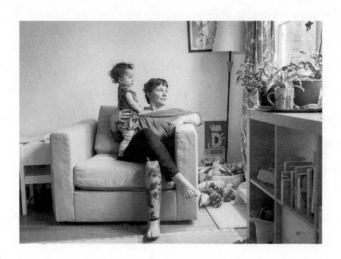

Christa Couture is an award-winning filmmaker, performing and recording artist, writer and broadcaster. She is also proudly Indigenous (mixed Cree and Scandinavian), queer, disabled and a mom. Christa's left leg was amputated above the knee when she was thirteen as the cure for the bone cancer she had at the time. In 2017, her article and photos on disability and maternity went viral, and she is passionate about the power of representation. Christa also often speaks and writes about grief, having lost two of her children as infants. Today she lives and parents her daughter in Toronto, Ontario.

Ricardo and Donna Thornton

from an interview with Eliza Hull

RICARDO

It was 1966, I was only seven, and suddenly I was placed in an institution by my family. At the time, this was common practice for people with intellectual disabilities like me. First I lived at DC Village, and then I moved to Forest Haven just outside of Washington, DC.

At the institutions, I found the staff hard to deal with. There were some nice staff, but most of them weren't nice at all. Being in an institution felt like I was doing time for a crime I didn't commit. It felt like a prison; the only difference was that there weren't any bars. I hoped one day I'd get out of there and just be like everybody else. I wanted that so desperately.

My older sister and brother were already in the institution. When I arrived, it took them time to accept who I really was. My brother didn't believe that I was his sibling. I wasn't close with them. I was able to leave the institution and go to my mother's funeral with my brother and sister. I didn't know what my mother's journey or struggle was, but I was grateful to be there at the end. I've never met my father.

My sister died in the institution. They said it was from a heart attack, but I think she died of an overdose of medicine. To control her, they would keep her drugged up like a zombie. It hurt. When she died, I told myself I would advocate for change. My hope was that nobody ever had to live in an institution and be segregated. It shouldn't happen to anyone. One good thing that came out of my time there was meeting Donna. To begin with, we were just friends, I was a fairly shy person and would mostly keep to myself.

As years went by, I was given the chance to work out in the community. At Forest Haven, you weren't allowed to control your own money. So, if you got paid for a job, you had to turn in your earnings. I tried to cash my cheque once, and they punished me by stripping me of my allowance. It was up to them to choose how much money I would get as an allowance, everything was controlled. To overcome some of those obstacles, we had to show them we could work, and that we are capable of handling money. They were preparing us to move out into the community. I was desperate to go to school so I could learn more.

Moving into the community was a challenge. It was a complete adjustment. After the institution, I was placed in a group home, that came with its own rules. Donna got a beautiful apartment. We both worked at McDonald's, and that's where I fell in love with her. I wanted to go and spend more time with her, so I went to her house for dinner. I missed my bus that night, and so I had to spend the night at her apartment. That's when she proposed to me. I said yes.

We had to follow a lot of steps; the first one was letting our social workers know that getting married was something we really wanted to do. They were totally against the idea. They said, 'You're both just getting out of the institution. You have no idea what you're getting into, just go to your group home and be happy.' We wanted to show that we could do it. It was tough pushing up against everyone's opinions, people really didn't approve. They thought it was going to mess up the system. But we just wanted to live like everybody else, or at least try to live like everybody else. We may not get to where everybody else is at, but at least we wanted a chance to give it a try.

We had a beautiful wedding, and there were people with disabilities in the wedding party. We invited everyone, and even asked the mayor to come. They didn't come, but *The Washington Post* did, and they reported on the wedding. Some of what they wrote was okay, but a lot was bad.

Years later, Donna fell pregnant. At one of her check-ups, the doctor told her that the baby had a problem. It wasn't moving, so they had to do an emergency caesarean. They called me and asked me to come to the hospital. I have always had a love of sport, and learnt to play basketball at the institution. At the time, I was playing basketball for the Special Olympics, and had a basketball game, it was my team playing. I remember I was told in the nicest way, 'You've got to go! You've got to be there!' They had to push me out the door. Luckily, I took their advice and went to the hospital; I am so glad I did because I got to see my beautiful son. I went back to the game when Donna fell asleep, and we lost! But I didn't care, because I was bragging, I am a daddy! Everyone I am a daddy! I was over the moon. We even named him after me, Ricardo Jnr, we called him our 'Little Ricky'. He was born prematurely, so he had to stay in the hospital for three months, until he was the right size to come home.

The hospital staff were nice, we had a social worker and she advocated for us, so that people didn't take advantage of us. She was a very strong advocate, when we couldn't do it ourselves.

Even though we felt supported, there were still a lot of questions from other people. 'Can you really be good parents?' 'Are you going to be able to manage?' 'Maybe you may want to think about putting him up for adoption.' And we had to convince and show them that we were capable.

There was an article in *The Washington Post* about the birth of our son that used disability slurs to describe us and our family. It was very shocking. So, we then had to come out and tell our story and show that our baby is a gift to us. And we're going to give our baby all the love we can, and for those who're negative about it, just watch what we can do. We had to stay focused, and we didn't give up. We had to educate the community, about how happy we were, as parents with disabilities. We make good parents; all we need is a little bit of support.

I was always playing basketball with the Special Olympics, so I found it hard to let go, which was hard on Donna. She would say, 'You have a son who needs you.' In other words, it took me a long time to adjust.

When he was a baby, we had to find people to help us. We went to a development centre for children and babies called Georgetown, which was a support system for parents with disability. They were very supportive. They were worried about Donna, and whether she was feeding the baby on time and clothing him properly. They helped us and talked to us. They showed us what to do, they enabled us to feel good, they made us want to be better parents. Because they taught us the skills, we were able to bring them into our home. I began being more present at home, and not just putting all the pressure on Donna. It took me a lot longer to learn, but once I learnt the skills, the proper skills of being a good parent, I think I carried the duties out very well. Not just being there for my son but being there for my wife. I loved when I really started understanding him, when he cried, I would begin to know exactly what it meant.

When we went to enrol him in school, the principal said, 'We don't have any spaces, we are full. We have no more room for your son.' We were shocked, so went to legal services and found an attorney that advocates for parents. He was enrolled the Monday morning after she came onboard. I don't know what she said or how she did it.

One day Donna went to the school with Ricardo Jnr, and all the other kids made fun of her. I had to take that chance to educate our son what our disability was, and not to be disrespectful, 'not to your mother who cares for you and carried you'. When Donna went back to the school, the kids and our son were more respectful. They accepted her. It was our job to teach our son that just because we have a disability does not mean you switch sides and you join in with the other kids. We wanted him to learn that Donna is his mama and I am his father, and we love him.

We always talked about disability to him, so he is probably

tired of hearing our story by now. I think he was about seven or eight when he fully understood that something was different with us.

I remember when my son would come home from school excited that he had homework to do, and neither of us could understand the homework. The teacher was fantastic in explaining it to us. We taught him how to write his name, write the letters. If we didn't understand the homework, there was always teachers willing to help. We might not have had all the tools in our home, but we loved him, and we did everything in our power to get support when needed.

I would read to him every night. I would also get him to read us a story. I never really understood what he was reading about, but every time he read, we all joined together as a family. Sometimes it was hard when we had to listen to his long stories, at times I thought I might fall asleep! Every time he finished, we would make him feel good and clap, we'd say, 'That's beautiful!'

He graduated from Calvin Coolidge High School in 2000. The teachers were incredibly helpful. We asked for extra help in finding out what he needs to do well. We're like any other parents – whatever we can do to help him, we do it. He has his own family now, is married with kids, and is very happy.

I loved seeing him grow up, and being part of his life right from the beginning. It's beautiful. We set a goal to get him through high school, and we did it. Often people didn't believe we could, but we never gave up.

I would tell any person with disability thinking about having children that you have a beautiful gift, and there are supports out there if you need them, don't carry the whole weight on your own, you're not alone. You can do it. You may get discouraged at times, but don't give up.

I want to see other parents with disability reach their potential. They just need to be educated and given the right supports. Now I am free, and I live my life the way I want to.

I have worked as a clerk at the Martin Luther King Jr Memorial Library for over forty years. I started at the age of thirty-two as a volunteer, and then was offered full-time paid work. My main responsibilities include sorting, stamping and shelving books as well as other clerical duties. One day I will have to retire, but I am not ready yet. I have travelled around the world with the Special Olympics and even met Nelson Mandela. I also have been to the White House and met many of the presidents and took my son along too. I'm proud that I advocated for change so that institutions were shut down for people with disability. Even though I have achieved a lot, my proudest achievement is my family.

DONNA

As a baby, I was raised in foster homes. I remember asking my foster mother where my real parents were, and she could never answer that question. In my foster home, I had brothers and sisters, but I was never sure if they were blood relatives. Because I had an intellectual disability, I had a case worker, and when I was about eight she advised my foster mother that I should be placed in an institution. I think my foster mother agreed because she found it difficult looking after me.

I met Ricardo at the Forest Haven institution. We became good friends. As I grew up, I was able to leave the institution. I had very mixed feelings about that. On one hand I was excited, on the other hand I was scared. *What am I going to do with myself? How are people going to treat me? How are people going to look at me?*

When I began transitioning from the institution into the community, I got a job at McDonald's, where I got to know Ricardo more as he was working there also. I liked working there because I enjoyed meeting other people. I was good at it, but Ricardo didn't like working there, he always said he wanted to go to school and learn more.

Together Ricardo and I would work for a half day and then go back to the institution for the other half. We had to give the institution our pay cheques and then they would give us an allowance. We didn't get to make any decisions; the staff made the decisions. When you're institutionalised, you have no rights, all choice is taken from you.

It was exciting to leave the institution, but it was also all we knew. We had to start again and learn from the ground up.

When I was finally able to leave for good, I got myself a job at the mall cleaning tables and housekeeping. I also got an apartment. Ricardo came one evening to visit, and that's when I proposed to him. I always wanted him to propose to me, but I took a chance and did it myself.

When we decided to get married, people tried to stop us. I remember saying to Ricardo, 'Nothing is going to stop me. We just have to keep on going. We are going to show them that we can do it.' And we did it!

Two years after we got married, I fell pregnant. We had a beautiful baby boy, who was two pounds, eleven ounces. He was tiny.

I loved seeing my beautiful boy's face when he first was born. It was like nothing I had experienced before.

Because of our intellectual disabilities, we had the media wanting to report on our birth, so we had a whole camera crew there. I remember when the cameras were switched off and lights were turned down, I looked at the doctor and asked him, 'Will my baby love me?' The doctor said yes. And then I repeated the question, 'No, but will my baby love *me*?'

When the media articles began coming out after I had given birth, they called my little boy a horrible name, I was so upset. He is a human being; he is a child: he shouldn't have been discriminated against. I just tried not to pay attention to any of it. I didn't believe what they were reporting. I didn't believe what people were saying.

At the beginning, I had to take on most of the parenting duties, it all fell on me. One day the baby kept crying; it was extremely hard. In the end, I just ended up crying with him; he looked at me and then suddenly stopped crying. Ricardo loved his basketball, and it gave him a lot of purpose, but I had to tell him that his child must come before basketball. Bit by bit, Ricardo got better at being a parent.

Together we loved watching our son grow up, seeing him smile. Seeing him play, developing and watching him grow. It's so beautiful watching them grow.

As a child, I used to tell him fairytale stories, and when he was old enough he would tell us stories too, and we would applaud after he finished. There was a lot of love in our home.

I am a hard worker, and I worked at Walter Reed National Military Medical Center as a housekeeper for thirty-one years. I recently retired, and they gave me an American flag to say thank you for my service. It felt very special.

My son is doing well. He is thirty-five years old now and married. He has three kids of his own, one boy and two little girls. His son has graduated from school. We are grandparents and we are so proud. My son always looks back and sees that his parents are doing okay. He calls me and checks up on his mum.

For any parent with disability, keep going! Listen to non-disabled people if you need support. Talk to other parents with a disability and create a community. No matter what, don't give up!

* * *

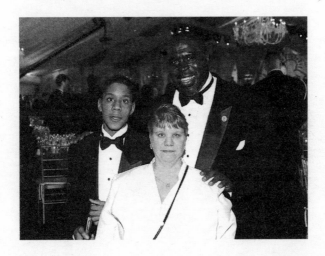

Ricardo Thornton is a clerk at the Martin Luther King Jr Memorial Library in Washington, DC, where he spends his days among books. **Donna Thornton** worked at Walter Reed National Military Medical Center for thirty-one years, but has now retired.

Ricardo and Donna are both active advocates for people with intellectual disabilities, speaking about their experiences and serving as role models, especially for young people.

As an athlete and ambassador with Special Olympics Ricardo has travelled as far as South Africa and Morocco. Closer to home, he has been an honoured guest at the White House, where he and his family met President Clinton.

Ricardo and Donna are proud parents to their son, Ricardo Jnr, or 'Little Ricky'.

Jasper Peach

Sometimes I don't think I've got this. I have nightmares where I'm underwater and my children are above the surface and I can't seem to break through. The worst ones are when they are the ones drifting away, only they don't know how to paddle up to the air, to the light and to safety. I have flashes of these dreams when they're in the bath. They're so happy and free, exploring how far the water travels in all directions when they splash; their joy is infectious, but the fears still flutter in my mind.

I'm forty now, but in my mid-twenties, during a perfect storm of stress and trauma, I got sick – and everything changed. After being promised that anti-inflammatories would fix it right up in a few days (spoiler alert: they just ate into the lining of my stomach), then going from GP to physiotherapist to rheumatologist, I was eventually diagnosed with fibromyalgia, and later chronic fatigue. Remembering this time in my life is really difficult – it's largely a blank: the memories aren't there to draw on. I was the sickest I'd ever been in a way I'd never experienced before, and I had barely any brain power at my disposal to process what was happening to me.

Trying to explain what my diagnosis means for me is hard. Old mate Google tells me it's 'a rheumatic condition characterised by muscular or musculoskeletal pain with stiffness and localised tenderness at specific points on the body'. But that definition doesn't describe how your friends disappear, or how you need to work out how to buy groceries when you can't carry the bags anymore, not to mention how terrifying it is to have unpredictable symptoms such as brain fog and wildly fluctuating body temperature. The strangest part of having fibromyalgia is that I can do many things just like I always did, but a few hours later – or the next day, or weeks afterwards – my body lets me know it was a terrible, horrible, no good, very bad idea. And that's the tip of the iceberg.

I don't like to talk about the specifics with friends, but rather give a broad brushstroke of 'all my stuff hurts and that makes most things difficult to navigate'. Their reactions are confronting. Pity, suspicion, eyes glazing over or the suggestion of yoga as cure-all are the worst responses. No, actually the worst is when people insist it's all in my head and if I wanted to recover all it would require is stronger willpower. I'd love to talk about the willpower it takes to face countless days in a row of severe pain, reduced work capacity and difficulty socialising, but something tells me the peddlers of these ideas aren't interested in hearing that.

After I got sick, I didn't think being a mother was possible. I cast the idea of having kids aside. If I couldn't really take care of myself properly, surely I couldn't take care of a tiny baby? But looking back, I see clearly that I *could* take care of myself – I just had to re -learn what that meant.

A few years into knowing one another, my partner, Tracey, turned to me and told me that having children was the meaning of her life. I was stunned – previously we'd always said that wasn't for us. Me for health reasons, her for political and environmental ones. We had just bought our first home, a funny little shack an hour south-east of Melbourne, and my immediate thought was *oh no, we're going to have to break up*. I voiced my concerns and said she would need to do that with someone else because I couldn't. I never wanted to keep her from her life's purpose ; I loved her too much. Tracey looked me in the eye and asked the question that changed everything: 'Will you think about it?' My reply came so easily and sincerely: 'With all my heart, yes.'

And so we parted for a few days and I got researching. I talked to my friends Jo and Quinn, who both have the type of pain I have and have each birthed two children. They described the experience of becoming a parent as healing. They said it was hard but the positives outweighed the challenges. There was even some evidence to suggest pregnancy removed the pain from our connective tissues, for a short time.

This became one of the defining moments of my life – realising that I could hold a belief and be certain it was true and then look into it and completely change my mind. The tide turned swiftly, and I bobbed along in the ripples that said, joyfully, *I want babies and I want to make them as soon as possible*.

*

So we had our babies. Tracey birthed them both. In the battle of who would give birth, she won the first round in extensive couples counselling sessions, due to her more advanced age, and I chickened out for round two because my body was protesting the idea of any additional pressure and stress. My limitations were clear, and I've always been better in the role of navigator than driver.

When the bone-crushing fatigue of having a newborn, then a baby, then a toddler, then a kiddo happened, it was nothing new to me. But my genius strategy of resting or saying no to things so I could function was off the table. You can't respectfully decline an invitation from your child to feed or jiggle them like you can turn down a festival launch. The choice is clear – it's time for a less glamorous life of scrubbing Rice Bubble concrete off a high chair or making a Play-Doh snail for my kid to eat or smash with her fist. Those moments of pure sensation that the kids lean into so wholeheartedly teach me so much. Have you ever seen a toddler pick up a rock in the garden and say 'wock, cuggle' while nuzzling the stone to their plump, ruddy cheek? Time stands still; in that moment nothing else matters.

It could seem like I wanted children for selfish reasons – that I wanted them to make me better. The truth is they do make me better, but not in the ways I anticipated. I am more compassionate, more generous and more focused. I'm exhausted and have more pain, but the love – the heart-swelling pride in seeing these rapidly growing humans make their mark on the world every day – eclipses everything.

Today, I watch my children learn how to navigate their

limbs. I see their minds expand and their skills develop. It's been the same for me, learning how to use my disabled body. I experienced a rebirth of sorts, involving frequent tears, eruptions of fierce indignation that I can't do what I want when I want, and eventually acceptance (with a lot of work).

I see my children getting to know their bodies and how they feel about what they can do. It gives me insight. I can be present with them through their worries, their pain, their confusion, because I know how lonely it can be navigating all this newness every day. Becoming disabled and becoming a parent both led to understanding how crucial humility is.

*

Some of my medications render me unable to tolerate direct sunlight (insert vampire emoji) and having two highly energetic cuties who will run onto the nearest road, into the body of water across the way or scale the side of a building to locate live wires next to open bottles of poisonous cleaning products makes it unsafe or impossible to go on outings without another adult present. I need to bring a runner along when we go out – Tracey bears the lion's share of that role.

I make up for my lack of speed and physical strength in other ways. I lather on sympathy after a tumble, point out the names of plants and can make up a song about most things. We each have our strengths in the parenting department.

My pain is unpredictable and can rain fire on any plans we are optimistic enough to make. A bad day brings everything to a halt and I tread water as best I can until I somehow regenerate some energy to get through, or until help arrives. I've found that when the kids need me, I can pull it from somewhere. But such energy loans are high-interest. On one particularly awful day, I was due to marry a couple (I work as a celebrant) in very hot weather, and in the lead-up had been dealing with some stressful and emotional life admin. The energy loan shark arrived the next morning in the form of a full-body migraine. I held on by my fingernails until noon, when the babysitter arrived and I could lie down in a dark room.

When I'm overstimulated, overstretched and overwhelmed, peace feels foreign and unreachable. Candy Crush, Netflix comedy specials (nothing with a plot), comforting chatty podcasts, and Messenger or WhatsApp chats are my come-down comforts. Then the inevitable Big Cry. Then a long, medicated sleep. And waking up with a delicious, warm kid in my arms, their sweet-smelling breath giving me everything I need to start the day. I know I'm back above the surface when I start thinking about what I can cook for my family. How I can nourish them and show them I care.

Because my disability is invisible and is a chronic health condition – and because my children are so young – they don't really understand it, but they're learning as they go, just like I am. I see us as peers – together we find out how to navigate this world that is excluding and disabling in some places, accessible and celebratory of diversity in others.

I identify as disabled, but for some reason I haven't said this explicitly to my children. Perhaps I'm waiting for them to have the benefit of a few more years' experience in the world to understand what this means. Being queer is a similar conundrum – in one of their books, *An ABC of Equality*, there's a page about gender and we have only just started having chats about that as a concept. When the right time comes, I know we'll be able to talk about disability too.

One of the hardest things is the price of disability. It costs many dollars each week to keep me upright and functioning as well as I can. Private health insurance, astronomical power bills (and the environmental guilt that comes with the heating or cooling being on a lot of the time), physiotherapy, osteopathy, acupuncture, medications, supplements, ad hoc babysitting when I need help on unexpected flare days, heading all over the countryside to expensive and stressful specialist appointments – these are all non-negotiable. They come at the expense of many other things, but the benefits outweigh the potential resentment. The financial and emotional budgeting is mindbogglingly challenging though.

Having an invisible disability means I need to remind people what I need fairly often, and that includes my immediate family. My needs change so frequently it's become quite a skill to identify them, and a deeper skill to voice them without shame. I'm still working on that. It's much easier to focus on the needs of others; it feels more important and sometimes more possible to meet the needs of anyone but me. But in our family *everyone* is number one. There's no contest, because if one of us is being overlooked, we all suffer.

At times my invisible disability makes *me* feel invisible, and in much of my life I've taken that on a bit too much: I constantly turn the focus onto the person I'm speaking with. It feels different in the disabled community — my crip friends online and in real life have a shortcut to understanding that makes things relaxed and easy.

The labour of being on a balance beam all day, deciding when to speak up and when to suck it up and get on with it is incalculable. My children have seen me cry on more than one occasion when the dam walls burst in private. I can tell them with age-appropriate words what's happening, but the most reassuring thing for them is to see that I'm okay and am able to dispense snacks at their request (both seem equally important). So I have to make smart decisions to keep the crashing waves from swallowing me up and knocking me off my perch of 'capable mum'.

I think all parents experience this, regardless of whether they're disabled or not. The pressures of the world we live in are immense and we can hide our emotions from our children and have them feel a change and not understand, or we can share the journey with them. Let them know what's happening.

On one occasion I had just emerged from a Zoom counselling session during a Covid-19 lockdown, and I sat on the couch having a quiet weep. Our eldest, who was three at the time, brought me a blanket and told me to have a rest. He then cheerfully got on with the business of smashing as many Duplo structures as possible. I was so proud of him in that moment, and proud of myself for raising an emotionally literate child who can identify what another person needs, offer it to them, and then move on to his own smashy, colourful pleasures.

*

There are times when it's clear I've got this.

Every morning I pick up a banana like a ringing telephone and, feigning amazement, say 'It's for you!' before handing it to one of my delighted, laughing children.

My son thinks chips are called Hot Chip Friday, because at the end of every week, after day-care pick-up, we call the chicken shop and order the big chips, the big wedges and the small gravy. This is our dinner, along with sour cream. Our daughter wears sour cream from head to toe, and our son drinks the gravy like soup. Everyone enjoys potato two ways. It's gourmet-adjacent, fun, cheap and easy. The chicken shop man says, 'Ah, Hot Chip Friday! Coming right up!' when I call in our order.

I have instilled in our babies a love of fashion and celebrating our bodies. In our case, fashion could be a box on your head and a single sock. But we take time to appreciate the creativity involved in colour and garment combos. Both our kids have been sprung giving their reflections huge kisses in the mirror.

We value kindness, courage, trying, laughing and farts. Our kids insist on helping with anything and everything. They feel proud when they can do something independently, but they have also seen their mum confidently and consistently asking for help when needed. Our eldest protested when I called day care from the car park, asking for assistance to get our wriggly toddler and her older brother inside safely. I listened to his words, his insistence that he didn't need help, and then warmly and firmly explained that for all of us to be safe and happy I would ring for help each morning until his sister could walk confidently just like him. That's exactly what we did, and after some time passed I was able to guide them both inside myself.

He has seen how the passage of time changes physical capacity at both ends of the age spectrum in our family. I'm mindful of being open to talking about these topics, which are so important for their understanding, and not just giving a blanket 'Mama needs help' retort. It's important that he knows his voice matters too, even though safety may outweigh his preference from time to time.

Our kids see their mums giving and contributing to our community – and receiving help as well. My mate Cat will often drop off a big container of food to make the week easier. Sherene will come over for a cup of tea and hold the baby for me while we talk. Heidi asks to borrow our son to play with hers for a morning when I'm home with both of them and Tracey is at work all day. The village is real and it's an exquisite honour to be a part of it.

I've got this – because I am the most amazing couch snuggler and TV watcher. I love to cook for my family (my nearest and dearest know I've needed a family to cook for over the past few decades so it's good I actually have one now). I talk to my kids about how it's good to cook with natural wholefoods, but I'm also cool with a 'that'll do' crinkly packet snack or squeezy yogurt pouch. One of my greatest joys is making apple boats for my kids. In summer we make icy poles from coconut milk and frozen fruit.

*

My wish is for our children to know contentment and fulfillment, and to be proud of who they are. I want them to have whatever they need, even if that isn't always what they want. Growing up with a disabled mum, they'll know different kinds of strength – resilience, courage to speak up, and saying no when necessary. But also saying yes to opportunities, and then expanding on that with the knowledge that they can always add caveats, contingent on the situation being fair and equitable for everyone.

I know they will know pain and hard work, because every human does, and perhaps they'll have an extended context for that, seeing their mums work together to make their lives as wonderful as we possibly can. They'll see their mums negotiating all sorts of situations on a daily basis, kindly and respectfully. Sometimes grumpily, because humans get grumpy. Being disabled doesn't turn you into an inspirational poster child, and being married to a disabled person doesn't turn you into a benevolent caregiver. We're equals who both do our best.

*

I hope my kids know that love is stronger than a body, and that a body that is in pain can love them with the strength and ferocity of a king tide.

Yeah, I reckon I've got this.

* * *

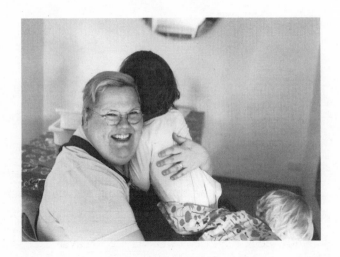

Jasper Peach is a broadcaster, storyteller and connector of people who sometimes works as a civil celebrant and always has too many projects bubbling away. They live in Central Victoria on Dja Dja Wurrung Country with their wife and two kids.

Joanne Limburg

When a psychologist confirmed that I was, as I'd long suspected, an autistic mother, my (non-autistic) son was nine. I held off sharing this information with him until he was thirteen, when he was given *The Curious Incident of the Dog in the Night-Time* to read for school.

'You know the boy in that book?' I said. 'I should probably tell you I've got the same sort of brain as he has.'

To which my son's response was: 'But you're nothing like him!'

'I know I'm not,' I said. 'Go figure.'

*

What was I like to him? What am I like? From remarks my son has made over the last nineteen years, I gather that I

- worry too much
- never shout

- smile too much at other people's babies
- am always dropping food all over the place
- shouldn't flinch anytime someone throws a ball at me
- go on about stuff
- don't look like me without my glasses
- am just weird.

Glean what you can from that.

*

Like many autistic people, I have a long narrative memory, so although I didn't know that I had been an autistic child, I remembered enough to know that my child was far more prosocial than I had ever been.

Many of my early childhood memories centre around objects or the environment: a pair of wind-up ladybirds, one red, one magenta; the very elaborate pattern on my grandparents' living-room carpet; the pear tree in full leaf that filled the view from my bedroom window in high summer.

I remember very little of people's faces. One snapshot that springs to mind is that of a row of great-aunts, sitting on chairs arranged in a row on that elaborate carpet: shoes, knees, handbags – and a twisting blur of smoke where each head should be. For years, I thought that the vagueness of this image must reflect the fact that grown-ups' heads were too far above my eye level for my memory to get the details down clearly.

I now realise that it was because I tended not to seek out

adults' faces, and I came to this realisation because my baby son couldn't get enough of them.

*

At some point, he must have realised that his mother's face didn't behave like most people's faces.

When he was about five or six, he would ask me, 'Why is your face like that?' This would usually happen when we were in the same room but my mind had wandered to a strange place, and obviously my face had wandered with it. My face does tend to wander off without my knowing.

Sometimes he did ask the question about other people. I think it was a five-year-old way of asking, 'What's up with them?' But he asked it most often of me.

One day, he was pretending to hate me, and I had to pretend to be hurt. He gave me notes, like a director to an actor: 'Show me the face of how that feels.'

*

My son kept watch on my face because children watch their caregivers' faces, and because my face sometimes did strange or interesting things.

I kept watch on my son's face out of maternal preoccupation (which is a fancy way of saying I thought it the most wonderful and compelling thing in the world), for the gratification of a shared smile and because I was an anxious mother who wanted to

104

make sure nothing was ever wrong.

And I have to concentrate on people's faces. I knew that, for some reason, I had to concentrate or I might miss something.

*

Small children's faces are generally easier to read than adult faces, and their speech is easier to interpret. Small children say what they mean: they want something; they don't want something; something hurts; something is pretty; they have a need; they have a question; they have something they want to show you; they have a complaint; they have a question.

I have never found it difficult to interact with small children. The problem is that, in order to be a mother, you have to navigate interactions with so many different adults: other parents; nursery schoolteachers and primary schoolteachers; health professionals.

The last can be particularly difficult. Autistic people – autistic mothers included – often approach a question by researching it. We prefer to find the correct word for something and to use it correctly. The problem arises when you come across the kind of professional who thinks that clinical words should be controlled like clinical substances, and therefore that if you, a parent, use them without being given them first you must be up to something – questioning their authority, faking a diagnosis.

I once mentioned hypermobility during an appointment.

'Who told you he was hypermobile?' someone snapped.

My cousin had; the after-school club leader had; anyone who'd ever seen him sit in a 'w', put his feet behind his head or pretend to dislocate his elbow in the lunch queue for a laugh would have agreed with them.

Perhaps the correct term for a mummy to use was 'bendy'.

*

Another set of difficulties autistic parents often report relate to sensory issues: smells, noise, the way that small children will keep touching you even in moments when you can't bear to be touched.

I'm okay with smell; I've been okay with touch. I always found crying very difficult. A tiny child's crying is designed by nature to be intolerable, and nature has designed it with precision. I feel a child's crying as if it were inside my own body, even when it's not coming from my own child. This is partly to do with noise – I can't bear raised voices of any kind, which is why I tend not to shout myself – but also because I feel the baby's distress without being able to process or filter it.

As my son once put it: 'When I feel something, it goes straight into you.'

But I try to keep a lid on it, for both our sakes.

Even though I do come from what a therapist once called an 'enmeshed' family.

*

I emerged – or failed to emerge – from that enmeshed family with a whole host of issues I'm sure have had an impact on my own parenting. Autistic is only one thing that I am, and there are very few characteristics I can identify as flowing directly from it. I have an upbringing and a history like anyone else. I have my happy memories that I want to reproduce for my child, and the traumas that I want more than anything to keep out of his way.

I know there are times when I got it wrong as a mother, but try showing me a mother – dead or alive – who didn't.

I complained about my mother when she was alive. My husband and friends complain about theirs. I've rarely met a person whose mother wasn't, in some way, a problem.

Autistic or otherwise, all mothers are destined to be impossible. We might as well accept it.

As my son was in the habit of saying as a toddler: 'Never mind.'

* * *

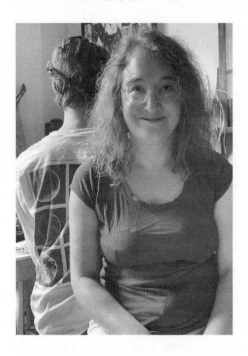

Joanne Limburg is a writer and creative-writing lecturer who has published a novel, three collections of poetry for adults, one for children and three nonfiction books. Her most recent book is *Letters to My Weird Sisters: On Autism and Feminism*. She lives in Cambridge, England, with her husband and son, and teaches at the Cambridge University Institute for Continuing Education. Joanne is a Fellow of the Royal Society of Literature.

Marjorie Aunos

The first time I met a mom with intellectual disabilities, I was a young twenty-year-old who knew very little about life apart from studying. She was just a bit older than me and already had two children. She wanted to meet me after hearing about me from her eight-year-old daughter, whom I was supporting at camp. When I entered her small apartment, she was busy trying to get everything ready for the next day, making sandwiches with baloney and yellow mustard, throwing in a juice box and an apple sauce. We talked for a good hour, and I was so in awe of her that I thought, *This is it: I know what I want to do for the rest of my life*. My purpose, my career – what would drive me for the next twenty-five to fifty years – had become clear. I would work with parents with intellectual disabilities.

As I completed my bachelors (undergraduate) program that year, I applied for my doctorate, convinced about the direction I needed to take to live a purposeful life. I read every scientific article published at the time, found an expert who agreed to supervise me and negotiated with my university. By September, it was done: I was going to write my thesis on parenting with intellectual disabilities and would start my career working with moms with disabilities.

At camp, many people had judged my pupil's lunches: what was in them, or rather what was *not* in them. But nobody had talked with the pupil's mom or considered that maybe fresh fruits and vegetables might be too expensive. That maybe she received aid from the local food bank, who offered non-perishable foods instead of fresh fruits. I heard judgement from them, whereas I saw resilience and love.

When I started my doctoral work, I was filled with passion and determination. I really felt and saw the discrimination and stigma these mothers faced. I saw the same dedication in the fifty moms I met in the following three years. Moms I sat with, had tea with, talked with. Yes, we did the official part and went through my questionnaires – but they also showed me their living spaces, talked about their children, even introduced me to their families and opened up about their struggles. I got to know them. They helped me understand what life was like for them, which was a totally different reality for me – a white, middle-class, well-educated young woman who was not yet a mother.

Even with these women's stories in my heart, I felt very alone. In Quebec, the province in Canada where I live and did my research, I was the only researcher in this specific field. Maurice, my co-supervisor, was three hours away in the neighbouring province of Ontario. We met often enough, when I needed guidance or when I had something to submit, but it wasn't the same. I felt like the only crusader, white-horse saviour, to these moms.

Nobody listened – truly listened – to them, and so I used my voice to make their needs known, which meant I needed to fight, argue, convince, demonstrate, advocate . . . every single day. The wall in front of me was made of child-protection workers (almost always), lawyers and judges (sometimes), professionals and community organisations (often enough) and even family members. All questioned their ability to parent – their capacity to raise their children. Intelligence seemed to have become a synonym of parenting for almost all of them, when truly, we knew – I knew, from my data and from those stories I had collected – that poverty, lack of accessibility, stigma and judgement were more responsible for the disparities we witnessed in these families. And it made me sick to think people were so quick to judge these women, when our society was to blame for the lack of support, universal accessible design and resources.

Every year I would attend a national or international conference dedicated to the study of intellectual disabilities. I started with a local conference down in British Columbia, where I met Gwynnyth Llewellyn and Sandy Tymchuk, two other trailblazers in the field. I was starstruck. I had so many questions, yet I also wanted to listen and engrave every word they said in my brain. They were my mentors, and they also knew of the importance of building a community.

From Victoria, BC, where I first met them, I was introduced six months later to some of Gwynnyth's doctoral students. I saw these Aussies as the community and friends who would make me feel less alone in my advocacy fight, and I was lucky enough that they adopted me from the get-go. To me, this was the consolidation of my purpose. In the last twenty-five years, we have met every so often, in Finland, France, South Africa, Australia, Canada, Norway, the United States, and the United Kingdom, our friendships growing and evolving as we did as humans, professionals and researchers. They were there in a South African hotel bar when I declared I would become a *single-mom-by-choice*. As scholars we argued about it, bringing forward the pros and cons of becoming a parent in this very unconventional way. But in my heart and soul, I knew I could do it because I had seen all these women do *single-motherhood* before me.

Deciding to have a child by artificial insemination was a big decision, one I took after a great deal of reflection. I was inhabited by all these women's stories, and I felt that if they did it within their living situations, I surely could too. I knew that I would probably not be discriminated against, and that child protection would not be called on me. I also knew I had the chance to choose the neighbourhood I wanted to raise my child in. I had a large social-support network, and I also had the means to pay for any extra help I would need. What I didn't expect or calculate is that things could rapidly change – it only takes one instant, doesn't it?

That specific moment for me probably lasted no more than five seconds. I was driving back to Montreal to go to work, while sixteen-month-old Thomas stayed with my sister and my parents in our family cottage. Black ice, a truck coming full speed in my direction, a car crash. I really thought this was it. The end of my life. I even remember thinking: *Today is a pretty good day to die.* But then I thought of Thomas . . . and how I had made the decision, and with it the promise, to raise him and be there for him until he was strong enough to be by himself, with his community of friends and loved ones. If I died in that moment, he would be an orphan. One that would be well taken care of, no doubt, but an orphan nonetheless. So I asked to live. His name was the last word I whispered in my heart and soul before the impact.

When I woke up, in the car, alone, with muffled sounds and unclear images, I knew something really wrong had happened. I was alive, but I couldn't feel or move anything below my neck. At first I thought of my legs, yet as soon as I realised my arms wouldn't move either, I panicked. And I begged – whoever was going to grant my request. I needed my arms . . . to raise my son. As a single mom, I felt I needed at least my arms to do that well. To not be too much of a 'burden' on others. To be somewhat independent in holding him and taking care of him.

I prayed. Only after my fourth attempt, when I had promised to make our lives be okay if my arms were returned to me, did I feel the twinkles in my fingers. This memory is as vivid as I am telling you. If the request was simple enough, the *making it okay* would be harder than I could have ever imagined.

Following a lengthy surgery to consolidate my spine, I stayed in the hospital for a month, half of it hooked to multiple tubes and machines in the intensive-care unit. In the first five days, I was in so much pain that I refused to see my son. By not inviting him in, I was saving him from the trauma, but despair was engulfing me. My ICU nurse was kind and gentle and caring, and she knew, from her twenty years' experience, that I needed to be reminded of why I had asked to live. She told my mom to bring my son to see me. Although this was what I needed, it was also the most gut-wrenching, heart-stomping, soul-crushing two minutes of my life. Thomas clung to my mom's shirt, trying to escape by climbing over her shoulder, all the while yelling as if the monster from under his bed had escaped to catch him. Underneath my tears, I told my mom to take him outside. She handed him over to my dad and said: 'I will bring him *every single day* to see you. I don't care if it takes weeks for him to get used to you again, I will make sure he knows who mom is. Mom is you.'

My mom and my dad did bring Thomas, every single day, after his afternoon nap, before his supper. He would come to hang out with *Maman*. At first my mom needed to be close to him, then nearby in the room, then in the doorway, then in the corridor. Thomas learnt the *new rules*: from his highchair, if he threw his wooden blocks onto the floor, no-one would pick them up for him. *Maman* couldn't yet bend over from her bed to do it. He learnt pretty fast that if he wanted to play with blocks, they would need to stay on his tray.

When I came home after an additional five months in rehabilitation, Thomas and I lived all crammed up inside my tiny house. I slept in the living room and had access to almost nothing in my house. I couldn't cook, or have a drink of water unless a glass had been left within reach on the counter. Doorways were barely large enough for my wheels, and even the door to the wooden ramp we had made was too heavy for me to open on my own. I was dependent in every sense, and I hated it. Thomas's bedroom was upstairs, so we determined that my mom would be my legs. If Thomas woke up during the night, she would pick him up and bring him to me. I would soothe him, care for him and make him fall back asleep in my arms before she would pick him up again to lay him in his crib. We did that for over a year, the time it took us to fight — tooth and nail — with the insurance company to get the new house I had bought with my parents (two apartments, one on top of the other) adapted to my needs: elevator, widening of the doorways, levelling the flooring, changing the windows and doors for better access, lowering the counters and cupboards, adjusting the bathroom.

I was so busy parenting, co-parenting, advocating for my rights, rehabilitating my body, figuring things out, that I didn't notice I was having a hard time being a disabled person. Up until that fateful day, I had been the most independent person I knew. My career had been central to my identity, and I felt I no longer could be the advocate for the moms I knew. I certainly could no longer visit their apartments, conduct assessments or support them in their homes, so what was left for me to do — to be? A mom — which I loved — but which I also felt I was failing — or rather, not attaining the way I had imagined I would.

All I could think was of those moms I served. All I could hear was that knock they received on their door. I knew child-welfare workers would soon knock at my door — for sure they would be. They had to be concerned about my capacity to raise a toddler on my own, while in a wheelchair, in an un-accessible house, in a body that was still foreign to me. At night I would make lists of all the concerns they could bring up: un-installed baby gate in front of the stairs, overflowing garbage cans I couldn't empty out on my own, cluttered rooms, medications easily grabbable . . . rambunctious two-year-old running in the uneven streets going to the un-accessible park (sand and wheels don't go well together). While I made those lists, I also prepared every intervention that I would put in place to ensure I would be seen and perceived as a *good-enough mother*.

Despite all of those sleeplessness nights worrying about that knock, no-one ever showed up at my door. Despite being a single mother, *scrambling to keep it together*, society had determined, without an assessment, without even meeting me that my son was going to be safe in my care. I was baffled. Yet I knew why. My living circumstances, the size of my wallet and the colour of my skin gave me the privilege to get parenting wrong, from time to time. It gave me the privilege of time . . . to get it right, to figure things out, without having to worry so much about being surveilled. I knew it. I knew of the discrimination *simply because of disability status* . . . and life circumstances apparently too, but felt I still couldn't speak about it, *just in case they would change their minds about me*.

Rendered voiceless by my guilt and the fear my son could be taken away, yet happy that he was still in my care, *no matter the reason*.

That fear and guilt, the loneliness, the lack of representation weighted heavily on me. I had friends and a community of loved ones who stayed with me and accepted me for who I had become, but did they *really* understand?

Through outdoor sports and kids' activities, I was also

meeting new friends: the parents of my son's friends. I was there at every soccer practice. Like any other parent. Not standing but sitting on the sidelines. My parents were there too. Because they wanted to be, as grandparents, and in case I needed them to push me on the mooshy grass that was hard to manoeuvre in my wheels. I was there tying Thomas's laces in the hockey room, even if it took me longer to navigate around accumulated snow in the adapted parking spot. I talked to kids; I spoke with parents. If they were shy at first with me, uneasy maybe, they warmed up rapidly. I am a social person. They saw I had the same aspirations for my child as they did theirs, although my son's soccer and hockey ability was undeniably non-existent.

I invited them to my yard for BBQ in the summer, or in my house several times, until one of them finally asked: 'What adaptations do you need, what can we do, to make our home accessible to you?' Until then, all of them had felt unsure of how to make it happen. This was the start of invitations and play dates. Parents would even come to pick him up and drop him off when they knew I couldn't. Making things accessible became a non-issue amongst us. I knew what to ask, and they knew what to do. They even learnt how to carry me up a flight of stairs. One couple even thought of levelling their backyard to ensure I could access it in the summer. Every single kid knew intuitively how to run around my wheels or knew to wait for me when I took them to see theatre and shows. Their parents trusted my driving abilities – or if they didn't, they never said a thing to me.

All this was different from the way I had imagined parenting to be, yet I was happy. Kids didn't really care about my wheels, it was actually sometimes seen as an asset to them. A perfect spot to drop their coats on when on outings, or to request a ride when their tiny legs got tired. They sometimes got concerned and would ask, 'How do you grab a glass from the high cupboard?' And Thomas and I would readily demonstrate. Either I took my grabber thing to get it myself or Thomas would show them how to put on the breaks, get on the footrest, onto my knees standing up to grab it for me.

None of them really questioned the why I was in a wheelchair until they were much older. They loved to 'test' if I *really* didn't feel it when they touched my legs. 'Close your eyes, I'll touch you on your legs and you tell me where.' Me being in a wheelchair was a non-issue for them. It might have made me even cooler than any other of the parents. What they seemed to care more about was how come Thomas didn't have a dad (and how that could that be). When this eight-year-old friend asked me, every person in my yard stopped talking. It was as if everyone had been wondering but was too scared to ask. And they were. They thought Thomas's dad had died in the car accident. When I told the story of how I became a single mom, I heard their sigh of relief.

Each year brought with it new parenting challenges but also, and mostly, a lot of joy. I was able to savour every little moment with him. I remember conversations with social workers and heath-care professionals. Telling me about their concerns about children of parents with disabilities. How unfair it was to them that they would *pick up the slack* and help out in the house. Children needed to be sheltered and protected. Their understanding was to bubble-wrap them. My son is well taken care of. He has learnt to make 'breakfast' at four years old. He could because the bowls were at his level and so were the cereals. That is all he needed when I was too slow to transfer onto my chair. He knew how to take showers on his own by that time too – I mean, I was beside him, reminding him to wash his toes or behind his ears, rinsing away the shampoo from his hair – but we no longer required Mamie (my mom) to do the steps physically with him like we had done for years. He also learnt young how to wash his clothes. I would make it a game: pick the clothes from the hamper, throw them to *Maman*, and into the washing machine. A little bit of soap and a press of a button. I was still the one deciding when we needed to do it, yet he could do it on his own – if he wanted (or remembered). I don't see how this would be bad for him. Despite knowing all of these things, he still remained a child. One that tries to convince me he has taken a shower, when *clearly* he has not. One that forgets to put some clothes in the wash because he decided to hide behind his closet door to change. One that asks me most mornings to make his breakfast for him. Parenting brings the same challenges as for any other parent, depending on the needs and abilities of our children.

Yet, because I am in a wheelchair, he also learnt how to be creative when buildings are not accessible. He is a first-hand witness to my parents and I working as a team. He understands the need for social justice, as he sees the disparities people with disabilities face every day – and it gets him mad. So much so that once he even asked to speak to the manager of a hotel we stayed at to detail everything that was wrong. A very shy kid — using his voice, like he had seen me use mine, to outline the obstacles and request for change.

My disability forced us to always think of solutions. We knew that if we focused on problems, we might be stuck in place, while if we made sure to always come up with solutions, we could go places. This mindset allowed us to travel to many countries together. Even if I was still unsure of the sound of my own voice after the crash, I continued to meet up with my friends in the field of Parents with Disabilities. I still had no idea that me learning to embrace my own disability was what would give me back my voice — strong from twenty-five years as a professional and even stronger from ten years as a mom on wheels. This is where I am at in my journey. A mom on wheels of a beautiful twelve-year-old son, I now know that I can use my voice to amplify the voices of all parents with disabilities. I do so by speaking about diversity and equity, bringing images of representation by sharing stories about my parenting from a wheelchair, and by bringing several parents together with researchers and professionals. My accident brought me to a much different place, but it made me stronger than I could have envisioned.

* * *

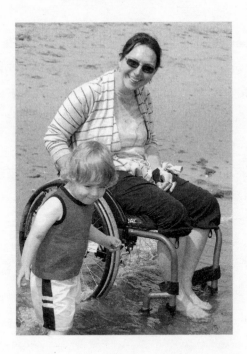

Marjorie Aunos PhD is an internationally renowned researcher, adjunct professor, clinical psychologist, award-winning inspirational speaker and member-at-large of the Council of Canadians with Disabilities from Montreal, Canada. She is the chair of the Special Interest Research Group on Parents and Parenting with Intellectual Disabilities (SIRG/PID) of the International Association for the Scientific Study of Intellectual and Developmental Disabilities (IASSIDD). She worked as a clinical psychologist and developed the first program offering support for families headed by parents with intellectual disabilities in the province of Quebec, Canada. In 2012, she sustained a spinal-cord injury in a car accident.

Marjorie believes that focusing on our strengths of character can lead to a fulfilling life. With her family she learnt to be a solution-finder to make her world more accessible. She is the author of *Mom on Wheels: The Power of Purpose for a Parent with Paraplegia*. You can listen to her speeches on her social media accounts and on www.speakerslam.org.

Jax Jacki Brown

'Do you want to have kids some day?'

I asked her on a cold winter's night, while we waited for a cab in Fitzroy.

Before meeting Anne, I'd never really thought about having children. As a queer wheelchair-user, I thought it would be too hard to conceive and, if I'm honest, I didn't believe I'd find someone who would love me enough to not only choose me as their life partner but have children with me. Internalised ableism meant I'd never allowed myself to entertain the idea that I might become a parent one day. So it was weird, only a few months into our relationship, to be asking Anne this question, letting it fall into the freezing winter air between us.

She responded right away – yes, one day she'd love to have kids.

After we'd been dating for four months, I took Anne home to visit my parents in northern New South Wales. While I went over to my best friend's house for a much-needed catch-up, my folks took the opportunity to quiz Anne about her intentions.

They asked her how serious she was about our relationship and whether she wanted kids with me. She tried to avoid answering but they persisted, asking if she wanted kids in general, even if not specifically with me. Eventually she said 'yes, someday'. When I got home, Anne told me what had happened. She was upset that my parents had forced her to have a conversation that we had not yet had together. I apologised for my parents' nosiness, and we agreed that if we were still together in a couple of years' time we would revisit the idea of kids.

I moved into Anne's place five months' later. Anne was basically living in my small apartment but her cats were getting lonely at her house, so we figured why not save on rent and make a home together? I brought all my rainbow things – my handmade queer pride flag and bunting with 'queers rock my world' stencilled onto it by a dear queer friend – and we hung them proudly in our home.

It was exciting to join our lives together intentionally. My parents built us the biggest symbol of our commitment at the time – a ramp into Anne's house. My dad is a hobby builder and had built me ramps into rental properties in the past, but this one was different – it was built to last. As it neared completion, Dad said, 'You'd better be serious about this woman because this is a beautiful ramp and I don't want to have to come and dismantle it.'

I was serious about her; after seven years with the ramp, we're still together.

*

Two years into our relationship, we revisited the kids question. I had been invited to speak on disability rights at an LGBTIQA+ conference. After my session, Anne and I went to one on 'Fertility Options for LGBTIQA+ People', delivered by the woman who would become our fertility specialist, whose name was also Anne. She spoke about the different ways LGBTIQA+ people could try to conceive. Dr Anne also talked through the options for testing embryos for genetic disabilities, and someone, not me, brought up that testing for disabilities and screening out those embryos found to be positive for 'abnormalities' was ableist and a form of eugenics. Instead of shutting down the discussion, Dr Anne said no one had shared that perspective before and that she'd be open to discussing it further after the panel was over. We stayed behind and ended up having a really great conversation with her. This experience motivated Anne and me to talk about starting a family – and before we knew it we were turning up to the fertility clinic for our first appointment.

We were both in our early thirties with no known fertility issues and a lot of excitement about this new chapter in our lives together. When we talked about how we might create our family, Anne surprised me by saying she'd love to do partner IVF and carry my egg in her womb. I wasn't really interested in becoming pregnant, but I liked the idea of having a genetic link to our child. Queer people and people with disabilities often have the legitimacy of our parenthood questioned, so knowing that my status as my child's parent could never be questioned was very important to me.

We didn't know any cisgendered men we'd feel comfortable asking to donate sperm, so we chose to use an anonymous donor recruited by our fertility clinic. We loved the idea that partner IVF allowed both of our bodies to play a part in creating our child.

*

At the information night for prospective parents run by our clinic, a nurse told us about the genetic tests run on donor sperm. For an extra fee, she explained, they could also run tests on us and any of our future embryos to screen for cystic fibrosis, haemophilia A, Tay-Sachs disease and two intersex variations – Turner and Klinefelter syndromes. Intersex variations are the 'I' in LGBTIQA+. Discovering that part of the community to which I belong – a community I greatly value – was being screened out was really confronting and distressing. We also learnt that all donor sperm in Victoria is pre-tested for cystic fibrosis, fragile X syndrome, spinal muscular atrophy and thrombophilia. We couldn't opt out of this screening: only sperm free of these conditions is accepted by IVF clinics.

Before attending this session, Anne and I had talked a lot about our capacity to raise a child – including, potentially, a disabled child. We'd talked about the barriers a disabled child might encounter, as well as supports and services they might need and advocacy work we might have to undertake as their parents to get them access to these things. These conversations forced me to confront my own internalised ableism. I feared

126

the additional prejudice and discrimination that a disabled child might encounter – I knew too well how utterly exhausting it can be. But I also knew that I could teach them resilience, pride and the value in being different, as well as connect them to the disability community.

So I told the nurse that we didn't want to be tested, that we wouldn't be screening any embryos. I said, 'Disability is part of human variation.'

In response, she leant across the table and grabbed Anne's hand, looked her in the eye and said, 'But it's *your* choice, is that what *you* want?'

It was as though she thought I had inappropriately influenced Anne's decision not to test for disability and she needed to let Anne know there was still time to make a different choice. I wondered, in that moment, what additional pressure the clinic would have applied to us to screen for disabilities had it been my body – my visibly disabled body – carrying our child. There is a fear of disabled people reproducing because we may create disabled children. Disability like queerness and other non-conforming identities are seen as not just 'other' but 'less than' by a society that seeks to reproduce the 'norm'. Disabled people, queer and trans people along with people of colour have long been discouraged or outright prevented from having children due to fear that we will taint the human race. The experience of disability, it is assumed, should be avoided, and that people with disabilities should feel ashamed of the things that make them different.

I am forever grateful that in my early twenties I stumbled

across the social model of disability: the idea that disability is not all these negative assumptions and stereotypes but is instead a human rights issue. Under the social model, disability becomes an identity, and to say one is 'disabled' is to say, 'I belong to an oppressed group fighting for my human rights!' I use the word 'disabled' here to reclaim it, not as a slur or a put-down but to explain that I am dis-abled or disadvantaged by an inaccessible society and other people's attitudes or stereotypes about disability, *not* my body or mind being different from a socially prescribed 'norm'.

Disability is a part of human variation or an aspect of diversity, but it is often not seen this way by the healthcare industry, and it was the multibillion-dollar IVF industry that we were entering to try to have our baby. It was very confronting for me as a political and proud disabled person to have disability framed as 'wrong', as something that should be screened out – for a fee by the clinic.

*

A few weeks later, we attended an information night for LGBTIQA+ folk wishing to conceive, and an IVF specialist gave a presentation about the services on offer. Someone asked how they could prevent disability. I was sitting beside her. The fear in the room was visceral: no-one looked at me while they talked about the options for screening. I was the supposedly terrible thing that could happen to their future children if they didn't do everything possible to prevent it, eliminate it, test for it, terminate anything deemed 'abnormal'. I felt invisible and hyper-visible at the same time.

Lying in bed that night, Anne and I talked about how horrible that moment had felt – for her, too as my partner. We asked ourselves why we stayed silent, what we could have said to challenge the narrative in the conversation – and what had stopped us from doing so. We concluded that we didn't speak up because it could have easily become combative, and it didn't feel like a safe space anymore. Considering having a child and investigating the ways to do so is an emotional and raw process for everyone. For people with disabilities, it can carry an additional weight of both internalised and external ableism. Sometimes it feels powerful to speak up and challenge people's views by providing an additional perspective on disability and at other times doing so feels overwhelming, exhausting and unsafe.

*

As part of undertaking IVF in Victoria, everyone has to undergo two mandatory counselling appointments at their fertility clinic, who then approves whether you can proceed with treatment or not. I was worried our counsellor would ask questions I didn't have the answers to yet, like 'How will you hold your child while wheeling safely?' But she didn't. She just asked us how we were going about starting a family and why we wanted a child, and gave us some documentaries to watch about donor-conceived people, so we could understand their experiences.

The counsellor told us it was important to tell donor-conceived children the full story of their conception early so they grow up knowing and it's never a big secret. We told her we were going to make a book about our journey for any children we had and asked her to pose with the two soft toys we had brought along, which were going to feature in the book. We asked this of all our specialists – the nurses, the embryologist, Dr Anne – and now we have a collection of cute, dorky snaps which document our journey.

*

For two weeks I jabbed a hormone-filled needle into my belly at precisely 11 pm. On the day of my egg collection, we arrived at the private hospital bleary-eyed for the early morning procedure. When I woke from the anesthetic, our specialist was beside my bed, looking sombre.

'We didn't get the result we were hoping for,' she said. 'I don't know why. Sometimes these things happen. We only got three eggs.'

This was a very low number for my age and didn't give us a good chance of success. I howled. This baby I now so desperately wanted seemed out of reach. I felt like my body had let me – and Anne – down.

We only got one embryo to the stage where it could be transferred to Anne – and it didn't stick. A few months later, we tried again. If this round didn't work, we would have to give up on the idea of having a baby. We couldn't afford endless rounds of IVF at $11,000 to $15,000 a pop. And emotionally the roller-coaster of IVF is deeply draining. It cost so much in part because we didn't have our own sperm so the system considered us 'socially infertile', which meant we were excluded from Medicare rebates for that first round. I argued with our specialist that lacking testicles and therefore sperm made us medically infertile as a couple but she was not amused.

In our second round of treatment, we got four eggs – three made it to day-three embryo stage, and each month we transferred one to Anne. We got down to our last embryo. The clinic transferred the embryos that looked 'healthiest and most normal' (in their words) first, so no-one held out much hope when we transferred the last one.

I was at a meeting when I got a text from Anne: 'I think I can see a second line, if I tilt it right and squint. I'm coming into the city to meet you and you can tell me whether you can see it!'

We met on a busy street corner in Melbourne, people and cars rushing by us as Anne pulled the pregnancy test from her handbag and we squinted at it excitedly. If you turned it at an angle and looked really hard you could, perhaps, see the faintest of faint second lines. We had to wait another day to test again.

The next morning we huddled in the bathroom and held each other. The second line was there and a little darker! Anne went for a blood test, and we waited anxiously for the call from the clinic. It came late in the day, which we immediately assumed was a bad sign – but it was good news! We got pregnant with our last embryo.

*

As chance would have it, we became pregnant at the time of the marriage equality vote in Australia, a strange and hard time to be creating a rainbow family. All the major news outlets aired homophobic and transphobic sentiments by conservatives. One day, wheeling down a back street in Fitzroy in the middle of the day, I just started to cry. I'm not a big crier; years of intense and painful medical interventions on my body as a child mean that I know how to hold my tears in, and when I'm in public I worry that any crying will be interpreted by strangers as me crying about being disabled. So the fact that I was wheeling along crying shows the impact homophobia and transphobia had on many of us at this time. I was also crying thinking about how our child would have to spend their life navigating ableism, homophobia and transphobia because of who their parents are, and I hoped I could bring them up to have resilience in the face of this.

Nationally 61.6 per cent of people voted 'yes' to change the *Marriage Act* and allow same-sex marriage in Australia. This means there are still a lot of people who don't think LGBTIQA+ folk deserve equal rights. Anne and I happened to be on holiday in my hometown when the vote was announced. Everyone was overjoyed and ready to party. While we were thankful that it had passed, we were also exhausted by months of having our identities and rights, and the question of whether or not we should be allowed to raise children, debated. Mixed feelings, to say the least.

*

Our lovely queer GP recommended an obstetrician and we excitedly attended our ten-week scan. I clutched Anne's hand and listened to the *thump, thump, thump* of our little love's heart beating as they wiggled about on the screen. After the scan, our obstetrician said she'd noticed on our file that we hadn't yet had any of the genetic screening tests and she wanted to assure us that it wasn't too late to screen for a variety of disabilities. She pushed a pamphlet across the desk at us. It outlined all the conditions they can screen for — Down syndrome, spinal muscular dystrophy, cystic fibrosis.

'Do you know what these conditions are?' she asked.

'Yes,' I replied. 'Some of my friends have them.'

The obstetrician asked, 'Are they still alive?'

'Yep,' I responded, 'they live full and happy lives actually.'

Clearly, her only perspective on people with these disabilities was one where the babies die or should be terminated.

At the twelve-week scan, the radiologist counted fingers and toes and told us cheerily, 'It's okay. They're all there.'

'We don't care if she's missing a couple actually,' I responded. I was thinking of my outlandish and accomplished friend who was born with one arm and one leg and how she would teach my child to be proud of any missing digits.

The radiologist just looked at me blankly.

*

At our twenty-week scan, the radiologist, without checking with us, took measurements of our baby. We assumed it was just standard procedure until she announced, 'Your baby looks normal, no markers of Down syndrome or spina bifida.'

*

I am pro-choice; I very much believe that people should have reproductive freedoms and be able to terminate pregnancies if they choose. I also know that disability is framed as a negative experience, a burden, something which should be screened for and terminated; *not* screening or not terminating is assumed to be an uninformed choice. Anne's and my desire not to know if our baby had any disabilities until they were born should have been respected by the medical professionals we were engaging with. Even in the delivery room when Anne was in labour, the midwife asked us – after reading our file – why we hadn't screened for Down syndrome. This ongoing pressure on us to justify our choices was exhausting and it also brought into focus ingrained assumptions about disability and the assumed worth of people with disabilities, which these interactions highlighted.

Before having our child, like any expectant parent I thought a lot about the kinds of things I wanted to teach her and the experiences I wanted us to have together. I wanted to impart to her that disability isn't a bad thing, just part of natural human variation. In those early days, when she was small and needed head support all the time, I tried all different kinds of baby carriers in the hope that I would find a way to carry her and wheel about, but nothing worked. They all pulled on my muscles too much and left me in more pain, and she would pick up on my discomfort and cry and cry. I wish I had been approved for my powerchair before she was born: it took ten months to get it and in that ten months I couldn't go out with her solo. If I'd had my powerchair, I would've been able to cruise about the neighbourhood holding her.

Now she's three and has just started a day and a half of kindy; she has friendships away from us and our little queer bubble. I have begun taking books with LGBTIQA+ families and characters with disability in them to read to the kids at her kinder. My wheelchair is a fascinating sight for the children, and books provide a keyway of connecting to it and understanding it.

We are not born with prejudices, we learn them. We need to provide children with the representations of diversity they can relate to and which frames it as something to find joy and pride in, not something to be ashamed of. My partner and I have done the peak queer parent thing and joined the Kinder Committee (queers love a committee) and we are assisting them with the ten-year plan for the kinder, so hopefully we will embed some LGBTIQA+ acceptance and knowledge of disability into the culture of the place. I use they/them pronouns and identify as non binary, so creating some literacy about gender diversity for the kids, educators and the parent group helps me feel connected and understood in my local community. My kid uses he, she and they pronouns interchangeably for almost everyone at the moment and doesn't quite get why some kids seem offended if she assumes they are a particular gender.

Nowadays, she spends a lot of time riding on my lap, about our house and in the outside world. She loves the feel of crunching over gravel or autumn leaves in my wheelchair. She knows the delight of finding a good hill to go down together. She is experiencing disability intimately, knowing the joy that can be found in moving differently in the world, and she doesn't view this as bad, or less than: just as the way I, her parent, does things.

Sometimes I still worry about my child having to navigate homophobia, transphobia or ableism in all its subtle and not-so-subtle forms, but we are doing our best to teach her pride in herself and her family, and resilience. And we surround ourselves with many fabulous queer and trans folks and radical people with disabilities, so that she knows there is value in existing outside the mainstream.

Recently she drew a picture of me – a circle with some stick-figure arms and legs protruding from it – and asked, 'But where is your wheelchair?'

Then she drew my wheelchair for the first time.

* * *

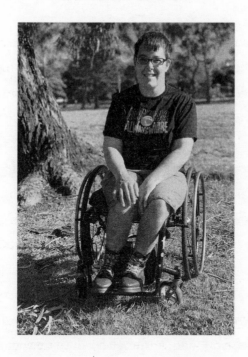

Jax Jacki Brown OAM (they/them) is a disability and LGBTIQA+ rights activist, writer, and educator. Jax's work has been published in *Queer Disability Anthology, QueerStories: Reflections on Lives Well Lived from Some of Australia's Finest LGBTIQA+ Writers, Kindred: 12 Queer #LoveOzYA Stories* and *Growing up Queer in Australia.* Jax is interested in how we can build resilience, pride and community for disabled people.

Daniela Izzie

from an interview with Eliza Hull

My desire to become a parent was thrown into question thirteen years ago when I had a spinal-cord injury and became a quadriplegic.

Everything changed in one day. I didn't want it to be my reality. I wanted to get better. For so long I kept pushing my new identity away. Of course, this was a natural response. A spinal-cord injury is traumatic. When you become paralysed, you have to relearn everything. It was frustrating and sad, and I mourned my old self. It's impossible to adjust overnight; it was a very long journey of acceptance; and understanding disability and what that identity means took time.

Three years after my injury, I started exploring disability as an identity more when I went to grad school to do a master's degree. I dabbled in disability studies, which helped tremendously. Knowing that there was a movement, and a community and history. It made me feel proud. Suddenly it became much more than just a diagnosis.

I had always wanted to one day become a mum, but when I became disabled, with my lifestyle, and needing as much assistance as I do, parenthood seemed daunting, like adding another layer of complexity to an already very challenging lifestyle.

I see my disability as like having a second full-time job as well as my actual job, so adding parenting to that seemed like a lot.

But then I met my husband, Rudy. The desire to become a mother came back, although the question was still there. How?

There was probably a little bit of internalised ableism, because I remember thinking, I can barely take care of myself, how am I going to take care of a child?

Finally, my husband and I decided we wanted to start trying for a family. We ended up going to see a doctor specialising in high-risk pregnancy, because I was concerned about my body's ability to carry a baby. Even though spinal-cord injury doesn't necessarily mean high risk, I thought that would be the best route because they'd be more knowledgeable, and I was right. I was so impressed by the breadth of knowledge they had about my disability, and the way that it interacts with pregnancy. I'd heard so many horror stories from fellow wheelchair, mom friends, about their experiences with different obstetricians, so it was such a relief to have a beautiful doctor who listened to my laundry lists of concerns and fears. I was able to let my guard down, and she was able to talk me through everything.

By the end of our consultation, she said go for it. It was so wonderful to have that support. She helped me give myself permission to make me realise I can do this. Then I got excited.

My husband and I took a couple more months after the consultation before we started trying. We made some modifications to our house first, including the kitchen, so that there was an island that I could roll under. We also created a mini cooking station because I wanted to be able to contribute by making food for the family.

Rudy was very excited to pursue fatherhood, but he was concerned for me. He just wanted to make sure the pregnancy was safe. I was also nervous about how he was going to deal with having kids as well as making sure my main needs were met, which aren't many, but it's still an obligation that he has every day. For example, he helps me get into the bathroom and gets me dressed. To be honest, we didn't really know what to expect.

In 2019, I got pregnant very quickly, in fact it was as soon as I went off the pill. In our first ultrasound at the hospital, they told us we were having twins. I was so shocked. I automatically started thinking, how am I going to do this?

I had finally talked myself out of the internalised ableism and had started researching how I was going to manage a baby independently. I was feeling ready to deal with motherhood. And then I was like, oh god, all the plans are out the window. Obviously, we were so happy above anything else. It felt so incredibly special to find out we were having multiples, like a wild gift. But I didn't really know how to plan for twins. I had nobody who was disabled to call and ask how do I do this?

In the end, it was good that I had initiated the journey with the high-risk clinic, because as it turns out, multiple pregnancies are high risk. They understood my disability and knew how to talk to me and treat me. I was very lucky there was never any negativity or discrimination.

They always spoke to me very realistically about everything. They presented all the risks and potential complications; some were because of my disability, and some were not. They took a lot of time to listen to me because I was dealing with a lot of anxiety. I was hugely fearful of miscarrying. Sometimes I have body spasms, and I would worry that I was hurting the babies. The doctors would reassure me and say, 'The babies are really well protected, the spasms won't hurt them.' Then there were a lot of questions I had that were very particular to my disability that the doctors would say, 'There's not really any research on that.' It was incredibly hard for me to let that go and trust that everything was going to be okay.

I was thirty-three weeks pregnant when we were suddenly thrust into the Covid-19 pandemic in April 2020. When I went into labour, I wasn't even sure if I was in labour, so we stalled at home for hours. Not knowing if I was in labour had actually been one of my main concerns, because of my reduced sensation.

We had to drive an hour away to get to the hospital, and by the time I got there I was very dilated, so much so that one of the babies was crowning. The hospital staff were worried that we were putting the second baby at risk, so they decided to do an emergency caesarean. The surgery would be a little more complicated than usual, because I've had surgery in the past which helps me manage my bladder independently. There were so many people there in the operating theatre. They had urology, anaesthesiology, and a team for me and a team for each baby. It felt like a loud community centre!

They gave me a spinal anaesthetic and I felt great afterwards. I've never had so little pain in my entire life. I felt better than I usually do!

After the spinal block, they finally let Rudy in to be next to me. He looked extremely scared. I remember saying to him, 'It's fine, I feel good.'

I could hear the surgeons consulting with one another. There were questions about how to manage the surgery because of the more complicated C-section. I enjoyed listening to them talk and hearing their professionalism. I was so in awe of what they could do. It was an incredibly positive experience and I feel very lucky.

There were parts of the birth that were incredibly hard, though. After the babies were born, I didn't get to spend time with them for twenty-four hours, because they were premature and they wanted me to recover, which to this day I still don't really understand why. During that period, I only got to meet them for maybe thirty seconds. They put them near my face, but it was just way too short.

After the twenty-four hours away from them, I felt so desperate and vulnerable. I so badly wanted them to be with me, it felt incredibly unnatural for them not to be with me. I think that was magnified because I am disabled, I felt powerless. There was no way I could just get up out of the bed and walk down the hallway and see them.

When I finally met them in the neonatal intensive-care unit (NICU), it was surreal, it really started to sink in, that pure joy. The desire to protect them. It was truly incredible. And that was the first time I got to hold my beautiful girls, Lavinia and Georgiana.

For two weeks, they stayed in the NICU, they were in a humidicrib, and I couldn't hold them. I was pumping milk, and we had to commute an hour every day to see them. We'd spend a couple of hours by their side, but it was never enough time. During that time, it almost felt like they weren't mine, like I was waiting to be a mother. At the hospital, there wasn't an accessible space to change them, so my husband had to do all the changing.

When we were finally able to bring them home, I was so relieved. It felt like all my anxiety slowly started to melt away. We were just so excited.

The first few weeks at home were fairly easy. Because they were premature, they just slept so much. The thing I found hard was breastfeeding. While they were in the NICU, they were given a pacifier to keep them comforted. So, they didn't develop their understanding of their mother's nipple. They just didn't quite know how to latch, which in the end affected my milk supply. It was so hard because I didn't get that skin-to-skin contact with them and the ability to practise it with them more. I also had a lot of trouble with just physically being able to get them latched.

Because we were in the midst of the pandemic, I didn't have the support I needed from a lactation consultant. I had no guidance. I kept pumping for six months, and occasionally I would try to nurse them, but in the end I did it mainly just to comfort them.

We had planned a lot around there not being a pandemic. We

were going to hire a night nurse to help us. But in the end, it just ended up being my husband and me.

After they stopped sleeping so much, we really went into survival mode. It felt like baby boot camp. It really was so much harder than I expected, but also so much better than I expected. Co-parenting has been tremendously challenging, particularly the way it intersects with my disability, with what I can and can't do.

I feel like it's taken us time to figure out our roles. As a mom, with instincts to do things certain ways, it's been hard having to communicate that to my partner, who might have different opinions, especially when you rely on that person for your own needs as well.

Ultimately, I just needed more support than I had, but we couldn't reach out for it because we were in the middle of a pandemic, so we went through some really hard times and felt incredibly isolated. My own mother also became disabled during the pandemic, so she also couldn't be as involved in supporting me. She's losing her vision very rapidly.

My advice to any disabled person thinking about starting a family with a co-parent is to find the right partner. Especially if you're someone like me, who relies on care, and this is not a reflection of my relationship with my husband at all. But when I was going through some difficult times with him, I thought my gosh, this could be bad. If he wasn't a good person, this could be terrible. I could be stuck in a bad situation that I can't get out of. And if I did get out of it, I'd get out without my children. In the USA, there's a couple of states that discriminate, where disabled people don't have equal parental-custody rights.

I believe when it comes to talking about the challenges of parenting with a disability, we need to have a space for it. It's emotionally difficult to share the challenges because I'm often afraid people will judge me or discriminate against me, like they will finally catch me out and say, 'See, you can't do it all.'

In the end, I pretty much just threw all the rules out the window. That's what I learnt that I needed to do.

At first I felt pressured to do certain things certain ways, because that's how people say you're supposed to do them. But then I was like, you know what, if this is going to work for me, I have to do it my way. For example, bed sharing. In the States, it's really frowned upon. But bed sharing is accessible parenting. I can't get out of bed; I am paralysed. So, it's the safest, most accessible option.

I am still bed sharing with them now and they're two years old. It's really helped with their attachment with me because there's many physical things that I can't do with them. But they really need that physical contact, and they need to feel loved; bed sharing enables both.

The girls are so caring and observant. I don't know if it's because they see Rudy being patient and helpful with my physical needs. They must be absorbing that, because they are starting to do things that I'm amazed by. I don't ask them to help me with my personal needs, because I don't want them to ever have to have that role. I want them to be kids and enjoy being kids. They don't need to grow up early. But they'll still do little things where it's their choice, because they want to help.

The other day, my foot fell off my footplate on my

wheelchair, and I muttered to myself, 'Damn, my foot fell,' and I was kind of groaning. One of my daughters ran over and said, 'Are you okay, Mama?' She picked up my foot and slid it perfectly back on top of the plate, making sure my ankle wasn't rolling and my foot was planted. It was secure and centred on the footplate, her attention to detail was absolutely mind blowing. I just didn't know that she had it in her, because she's only two. So, so kind.

They absolutely love interacting with my chair — it's their jungle gym. They climb all over me!

They can't climb on the spokes on the wheels, because then I can't roll anywhere. I'm literally stuck. But I secretly love it.

I'm always taking them for rides. We absolutely love it. They think that everything with wheels is a wheelchair. They thought the other day that the grocery cart at the store was a wheelchair. It's very cute.

It's been so amazing watching them grow. It's just brought us so much joy. I have gone through so many struggles and so many difficult times, and they've brought so much lightness back in my life.

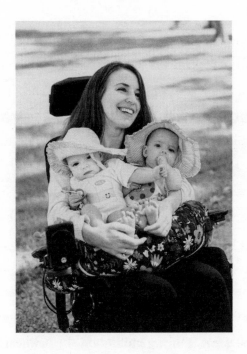

Daniela (Dani) Izzie is a disability advocate and wheelchair user, and a new mom to twins. She works full-time in social media and advertising within the wheelchair industry. She holds a master's in English literature with a focus on disability studies. As an advocate, her work centres on elevating voices of disabled parents, and she is the subject and producer of *Dani's Twins*, an upcoming documentary about pregnancy and motherhood as a quadriplegic during the pandemic. A dual citizen of the United States and Italy, she now lives in rural Virginia with her husband, kids and trusty service dog.

Oscar and Estefani Arevalo

from an interview with Eliza Hull

Oscar: As a young baby, I had a high temperature which caused me to become Deaf. During childhood, I used hearing aids and had to learn to lip read. My parents were incredible, though, in enabling me to learn American Sign Language.

I live in Bakersfield, California, where there is a very small Deaf community, and I met Estefani at Deaf church. We dated for six months and quickly fell in love. Within seven months, we were married. I always wanted to be a father, but we took our time. While she studied, Estefani and I got to know each other, and we got a dog.

In 2017, two years after living together, Estefani became pregnant with our beautiful daughter, Everlyn. Luckily there weren't any complications with the pregnancy, and she went to full term. The birth went incredibly well too. At times I did worry about how we were going to manage with a newborn. I would often wonder how we would know our baby was crying. It helped that we researched a lot and found an alarm which vibrated whenever the baby cried.

Estefani: During the labour, we had an American Sign Language interpreter, but they left shortly after the birth to go home and rest. We weren't expecting the doctors to come in, but they wanted to conduct the hearing screening test. Oscar had just had a brand-new cochlear implant inserted, so he wasn't able to understand what they were talking about during the screening. Our baby was crying and was being fussy, and I was sleeping as I was so exhausted after labour. After I woke up, I asked Oscar about the outcome of the hearing test. 'I don't know,' he said. 'I didn't really understand what they were saying. They said they're going to reschedule for the next two weeks.' And I remember thinking, okay, that's weird. I assumed they mustn't have been able to do the test, so I let it go. We were both just so incredibly thrilled to have a beautiful new baby. We were just focused on her, taking care and adoring our new child. The excitement really was palpable.

Two weeks later, we were due to go to our next hearing screening test, but our sleep schedule was off, and we were all exhausted, so we postponed the appointment. Two months later, I started noticing that our baby was super quiet, she was just always so serene and didn't cry as much as I assumed a baby would. If we made sounds, or even if the dogs barked loudly, she would still sleep very peacefully. It threw me off, and I started to wonder, could she be Deaf? I called the hospital and scheduled another hearing test. Weeks later, we had the appointment, and ten minutes into the appointment, the nurse looked worried and said, 'I just want to let you know that your daughter has failed the hearing test.' I remember saying, 'What?' I was shocked. We didn't mind if our chid was hearing or Deaf, but to be honest we always expected they would be hearing because we didn't know of any generational Deafness in our family. Then they added, 'What do you mean, you knew that didn't you? She failed the first time just after she was born.' It became obvious that my husband had missed it.

Oscar: I hadn't understood what the nurses had said because I didn't have an interpreter present, they didn't even have an interpreter on video for me to be able to communicate. They had assumed because I had the cochlear implant and I am hard of hearing, that I would be able to understand. It was incredibly frustrating. They really should have waited to test our daughter when an interpreter was present. Because I speak, they just assume that I can hear.

Estefani: At first my parents didn't believe that our daughter was Deaf. They didn't think it could be genetic, because we don't have anyone who is Deaf in our family. My mother gradually accepted it, but it took my father longer. He would visit us and often talk verbally with my daughter. As she got older, she started signing more, and my father finally accepted that she's Deaf, and learnt a bit of sign to be able to communicate with her.

Oscar: My parents are not Deaf either. But they were very supportive when they found out our daughter was. They were just happy she was healthy and happy. They also felt that she would benefit because we're both Deaf and therefore would know her needs.

Estefani: We fell pregnant with my second child, a beautiful baby boy named Jabez, two years later. Eighteen weeks into the pregnancy, my waters broke, but luckily I made it to full term, all the way up to forty-one weeks. Because of all the complications during the pregnancy, we had a lot of appointments, and for the most part we were provided with an interpreter in person or via video. But during one appointment there was a new doctor who said he had never had a Deaf parent before and that it was our job to find and pay for an interpreter.

Oscar: We had to educate him about the *Americans with Disabilities Act*, that it's our right to have an interpreter and be able to communicate freely. Still today many people don't know that. Often it feels like we spend so much time having to constantly educate others about our rights as Deaf people. It can be extremely exhausting.

After my son was born, he had his hearing test; for his we were given an interpreter via video. His results came back inconclusive, so they asked to reschedule.

Estefani: When they were testing him, they seemed extremely worried. I had to reassure them: 'I have a Deaf daughter. I'm not worried.' The doctor just ignored me and said he may have fluid in his ears, so we should massage them, and then they suggested we test again in two hours' time. I knew because of our newfound generational Deafness that he would be Deaf. When they came back to test again, they were initially very apologetic, they began to look sad and worried. Then they said, 'He didn't pass the test, we will need to refer you to an audiologist.' I said, 'Okay, that's fine.' I was just quiet and expressionless. I think the doctor was really confused and confronted by my reaction. They assumed I would be upset that our boy was hard of hearing.

Oscar: That's one of the problems. People always assume that we're sad that we're Deaf. People think that our Deaf children won't have a normal life. It's such a misconception. I have a cochlear implant and I wear it. But I disagree with implanting babies with them. For one, it's not always guaranteed that they'll be able to use it for their whole life. Half the people that I have met that have had their kids inserted with one usually don't use it. So, it doesn't always help them, and it doesn't benefit their lives very much. Also, a lot of children that have cochlear implants miss out on learning sign language. What's important is that you have language and you're able to sign and communicate. For us as a family, sign language is a very crucial part of our existence. Ultimately, I want our children to have choice, and if they choose to have a cochlear implant when they're older, that's fine. I don't want to force it on them when they are not part of that decision-making. I will support their decision with whatever they choose. But they would have to really show us that they want to use it, and not just use it one day and not the next.

Estefani: There is such a mentality that to be Deaf is a deficit. People often think that our children can't succeed. Audiologists automatically suggest our children should have cochlear implants, as though they need to be fixed. The thing is, once a cochlear implant comes off, they're still Deaf.

My children are fine, they have very happy lives. Normal lives. They play, have baths, eat well. And we have sign to communicate. They love music and feel it through their bodies. As a family, we have a beautiful life.

The hardest part is the challenges we face in society, because we live in an inaccessible world where Deaf people are not given the chance to communicate freely. Just yesterday I had to take my son to the hospital because he had a cough that was bothering him. I had an interpreter on video, so the appointment was going really smoothly. We then had to get some more testing, and while we were waiting, I started to communicate with another patient who could use some basic sign language. The doctor saw us communicating. When they called me back to see the results of the X-ray, they asked the other patient to come in and interpret for me. I was taken aback. 'Wait, no,' I said, 'we have the video system we can use.' They said, 'What's that? No, this person can interpret for you.' They were trying to tell me that the results were fine with their thumbs up. But I had more questions I wanted to ask, I felt limited in my communication. And the other patient clearly looked stressed. I didn't want this stranger knowing private information about me, it violates patient confidentiality. After I pushed back, the doctor rolled their eyes, saying that everything was fine. I just couldn't believe it.

In our home, it's a lot easier, and we use American Sign Language 100 per cent of the time. The kids also watch TV programs that are in ASL, sometimes we use captions as well.

We have always wanted our environment to be as Deaf-friendly as possible. My little boy is five months old now, and he is already signing 'Mama'. He's picking up so much, when I sign in front of him, he understands. My daughter is three going on four now, and she signs all the time, she's an incredible communicator.

Since having kids, we have learnt ways to adapt, for instance when we want to make an appointment for the kids, we use video. There's an app that I press on my phone, and it calls and connects with someone who can use sign language. It's a great resource because they then relay the information we need. We also use cameras and have baby monitors that keep an eye on the kids as well, so we can always see them. We use a lot of visual technology.

A lot of people feel sorry for us because we are Deaf. People have even said that we shouldn't have had babies, because we have genetically passed down our Deafness. What they don't understand is that I am very happy that I have Deaf babies. I'm not sad in the slightest. People say, 'Don't you want them to be fixed? You should get cochlear implants for them. Don't you want to hear? Don't you want to use your voice and speak?' I just reply, 'No, I don't want to.' People don't understand Deaf culture, they don't understand our life. I would love my children if they were Deaf or if they were hearing. It doesn't matter.

Oscar: A lot of people have very closed minds. They don't understand where we're coming from. People generally focus on the medical side of things, with the assumption that we ought to be fixed. They focus on what's not working, instead of opening their minds to how we live – with Deaf culture, with Deaf people, in a Deaf community – and how happy we are.

Estefani: As a child, I was very good at sport, but I was constantly told that I couldn't participate. I was left out of school activities often because of communication barriers. It made it hard communicating with my classmates. I remember going to prom and they didn't have an interpreter there, I felt incredibly alone. That's not the life I want my children to grow into. Due to both of us going to a hearing school, where there was only a small Deaf program, we are adamant that our children will go to a Deaf school where they can freely communicate with each other in their language. Learning from the past, we now know what's best for our children. While the nearest Deaf school is three hours away, we are willing to make the move.

My kids bring me so much joy, I love teaching them sign language, I just am so incredibly grateful to have them, I love watching them grow and learn and use more sign language as a family. I want them to access a school that is like their home, inclusive and accessible.

Oscar: Having seen what a lot of Deaf kids go through in hearing schools, a lot of them don't have the right resources to help them navigate life, even after finishing school. I played basketball in high school but was stuck on the bench a lot of time. I don't want that for my children. I want them to be included. I want them to have the opportunities to be involved in anything they want to do.

I love when I come home from work at the end of the day, and they are so happy to see me. My daughter signs 'Dad' and then hugs me tight. It just brings me so much joy.

Our hope is that we create a home, and a community where Deaf culture is central to our children's lives. We want them to live in a world where communication is easily available. Where they have equal access to communication wherever they go.

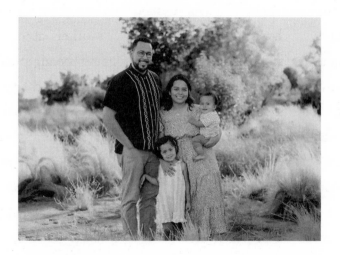

Estefani Arevalo is a content creator. She loves making content about sign language for kids, and has a large following @thatdeafamily on Instagram. She has two Deaf kids and loves to teach them American Sign Language.

Oscar Arevalo is a master automotive technician. He loves to learn new technology and spend time with his kids.

Debra Keenahan

'Mrs Keenahan, there is a problem with the baby ... she has dwarfism.'

This is how a doctor told my mother about my achondroplasia, when I was three days old. Achondroplasia is a genetic condition that can be passed on to a child if a parent has the condition. But it can also occur spontaneously, as it did with me. Both my parents and four brothers were average height and there was no record of the condition occurring previously in any branch of our family tree. To this doctor my dwarfism was a 'problem', but to my parents I was simply their baby girl who they loved with all their hearts.

Dad was determined that I would not be deprived because of my disability. He and the rest of my family resisted any attempts to separate me from the wider world.

Throughout my childhood I saw medical specialists to prevent secondary complications, such as bowed legs. In 1962, the medical thinking was that this was the result of a normal-sized torso pressing down on short legs. Intervention at that time required that at puberty my legs be broken, straightened and reset. This painful procedure would take twelve months and success could not be guaranteed. I did not have these operations because my family prevented my legs from bowing by carrying me throughout my toddler years. Having older brothers made this easy. Many different techniques were used to ferry me from place to place. I remember being 'a bag of coal' slung under one brother's arm, my legs dangling forward and my head getting a view of where I'd been. Another brother always held me as if I was sitting in a chair – then I could see where I was going. I had many different visual angles of the world. My memories of my mother from that time are of being cradled and rocked in her arms. When my third brother crossed his legs when he sat on the lounge, I would sit on his crossed leg and he would swing me for what seemed like forever. He also taught me how to draw. I would wrestle with my fourth brother. I took pride in once splitting his lip when he was tormenting me; he was too slow to get out of the way of my swift, tiny-fisted uppercut. I was always able to hold my own with my brothers – which stood me in good stead when I became a parent myself.

I found out I was pregnant when I was thirty-eight. A cascade of emotions washed over me – shock, joy, wonder, apprehension, delight and awe. I had wanted a child for seven years. Having given up on having my own, I had started the adoption process. Now I put those documents aside and commenced a silent mantra: 'Please let it be a little girl, please let it be a little girl, please let it be a little girl.' There were practical reasons for my gender bias. I was going to be a single parent and I thought it would be simpler for both myself and the child if we were the same sex. Particularly when it came to puberty. The thought of dealing with a bolshie teenage boy who could potentially be six foot tall was quite daunting. Because just as there was a 50 per cent probability we would share the same sex, there was a 50 per cent probability the child would be average height. My child's father is average height and with my genetic profile, in which the gene for achondroplasia is dominant, that percentage is well established.

Although I used the word 'little' in my mantra, I actually didn't mind if the child had dwarfism, because I never considered my physical being a 'problem'. I always say that my dwarfism doesn't disable me, what disables me are people's attitudes to my dwarfism.

Unfortunately, this was illustrated when I attended my first appointment with the gynaecologist to whom my GP referred me. Apparently, this gynaecologist had experience working with dwarf mothers. After the cursory introductions, he read my doctor's notes: the ultrasound clearly established the foetus had achondroplasia. He looked at me and said matter-of-factly, 'You should have come to me earlier. I could have done something about this.' There was no doubt what that 'something' was.

I have since often wondered how he counselled other women who were pregnant with dwarf babies, or who were single mothers. Or was his concern only because I was the trifecta – a dwarf woman, pregnant with a dwarf child, choosing to be a single parent?

My dear friend, who had come along to the appointment as my support person, reassured me I had neither misheard nor misunderstood the specialist's words, or the intent of his message. We said nothing as we walked to the car after the consultation. She opened the door for me and once she was behind the wheel, turned to me and said – 'You want to cry, don't you?' My tears flowed. I was simply gutted. My friend was irate. It was yet another occasion when a harsh moral judgement was unthinkingly cast without care or consideration for the weight of the words on the recipient.

The gynaecologist's declaration about my unborn child seemed like a cruel echo of the doctor's pronouncement to my mother when I was just days old – suggesting little has changed in attitudes towards people with disability.

When I fell pregnant, I knew my mum was dying, so I had requested to have my baby's sex identified during an ultrasound. It was that ultrasound that also identified she shared my dwarfism. I told Mum as much as possible about her grandchild before she died – including her name: Sarah Elizabeth. Elizabeth was Mum's middle name. I was also able to tell Mum that the baby would be small, like me. Mum responded to that news with the most beautiful, gentle smile – I can still see it in my mind's eye.

I was also excited to share the news from the ultrasound with Mum's friends, but I wasn't able to tell them about her smile because after I'd told them the baby had my dwarfism one of Mum's friends leant forward, placed her hand on my forearm and enquired with concern, 'Does that disappoint you?' I turned and walked away.

My response to that question was totally visceral. My heart pounded so loudly its pulsing resounded in my ears. I remember looking down, needing to be mindful of my footing.

I felt like a deer in headlights. I sought privacy in a toilet cubicle. I was experiencing a torrent of emotions – shock, great hurt, a deep sense of betrayal – but then as I had learnt from having experienced far too many such mindless attacks (and I purposefully choose such a strong description), when I calmed my breathing my familiar, resolute determination came back. Under such attacks, I become determined that I will be the best I can be at whatever it is assumed I am incapable of doing or being because I have dwarfism.

My parents never considered me a disappointment. The shock, hurt and betrayal I felt at being asked that question – which made me realise that person must have always judged me to be 'less than' others – was as much on Mum's behalf as it was for myself. As I regained my composure, I resolved to be as good a parent to my child as Mum was to me. Which meant my daughter would always feel loved and accepted and I would endeavour to give her the best foundation possible – a strong sense of dignity. What I wanted for my child is that she would value herself and not tolerate anything less than respectful treatment from others – which is what all people deserve.

My desire for Sarah to have a strong sense of dignity was borne from a lifetime of experiences in which I had learnt to navigate social situations and peoples' responses to my physical difference so that I could complete sometimes even the most mundane of activities.

From my own parenting, I knew food would always need to be on the table, I'd have to soothe her after scrapes and tumbles, and there would be many stories to read (a very important practice in our household), homework to be monitored and innumerable other practicalities. But my parents had also taught me that a child's emotions – particularly how they feel about themselves – and how the child treats others are perhaps a parent's greatest responsibility. If I wanted Sarah to grow up only accepting respectful treatment from others and treating others the same way, I knew she needed to see me behaving that way – and I knew that because of our dwarfism, there would be many instances when my resolve would be tested.

Children are naturally curious and are constantly learning about the world and the people in it. It is one of the responsibilities of parents to guide them through this process. How effective parental guidance is in challenging situations can have a significant impact on more than just the child. In particular, how parents manage their child's curiosity about those who look different from the majority can shape the child's attitudes towards and treatment of people with disability. As a parent with disability and the parent of a child with disability, I knew I would need to model to my child how to manage the vast spectrum of responses her physical difference would garner from children and adults alike. But it is particularly challenging when it is necessary to manage 'careless parenting' by another parent.

One day on my lunch break, when I was waiting in line for an available teller in a bank branch, a mother with a young son no older than four walked in and joined the line directly behind me. The young boy acted like many children do when they see someone with dwarfism: by immediately expressing amazement that an adult was not much bigger than him. He made the innocent enquiry, 'Mummy, why is that lady so small?'

Without hesitation, this boy's mother delivered the following explanation in such a vociferous manner it drew the attention of all the customers and tellers. 'I'll tell you why she's so small! She didn't eat her dinner! So, if you don't eat your dinner, you'll grow up to look like that!'

Now, it may be that this mother, anxious to meet her responsibilities in monitoring the physical wellbeing of her child, was having a bad day and jumped at an opportunity to modify her child's behaviour. But such careless parenting can have far more harmful consequences that an uneaten meal. In response, I turned around and stated earnestly but I hope not as loudly, 'Excuse me! I have done nothing wrong, and neither did my parents.' I then addressed the boy directly, trying to speak in a more conciliatory tone. 'Young man, I have dwarfism. I was born this way – small. And I always ate my dinner!'

I turned and walked out of the bank without completing my transaction. I took a few deep breaths once I was in the privacy of my car, then returned to work.

Although my daughter was not with me on this occasion, I knew I would need to prepare her for managing such situations. Careless statements and actions often present as negative judgements about our very being and can feel like attacks on our self-esteem – and negative ideas and attitudes about those who are different can all too readily be communicated too. A parent's responsibilities extend significantly beyond considering the physical requirements of our child: they also encompass guiding them in how to behave towards others.

It is a great relief, and even cause for minor celebration, when we are the subject of much more careful and thoughtful parenting. On one such occasion, we were enjoying a family day out at the beach with our two puppies. Needing to use a public toilet, I left Sarah, who was eighteen at the time, outside with the pups. While I was inside, a young boy, maybe three or four, and his mother approached the toilets. On seeing Sarah, the boy expressed astonishment at standing eye-to-eye with an adult. Apparently, he found Sarah far more interesting than the puppies and proclaimed as much to his mother. As the pair entered the toilet block, I had finished drying my hands and was walking down the corridor towards the exit. When the boy saw me, he stopped still with such a look of amazement on his face I didn't think it was possible for his eyes to get any bigger. With his hands in the air for emphasis, he said, 'Mum! Why are there so many of them?' I couldn't help but smile broadly as I met the mother's eyes, and she smiled back.

I assumed the boy had seen Sarah outside, and she confirmed as much when we met up. As Sarah and I were smiling about the boy's words, the young family exited the toilet block. Seeing us, the mother guided the young boy over. She immediately apologised if anything he said had hurt us and told us she had explained to him that all people are different – some are big, some are small, sometimes people can be much bigger than many others and sometimes people can be much smaller. We happened to be much smaller, but everyone should be treated the same.

We reassured her that we were not hurt or offended and in fact very much appreciated the way she handled the situation.

We spoke only briefly to the boy, because by now Sarah and I were just part of the scenery for him: there were two puppies to play with and they were far more interesting.

*

I wanted Sarah to grow up with dignity and self-respect which she could rely on to nurture herself and guide her through situations in which she would have to assert her right to appropriately respectful treatment. Sarah was aware from a very young age that she and I were physically different from others; she learnt this from seeing people's reactions to me. But interestingly she told me recently that she has never thought of us as short – especially when we're at home. It is only when she is out that she is made aware of her dwarfism.

*

On a family outing to a parkland area, we encountered an example of careless parenting. When we got out of the car, another family in the car park found our dwarfism such a source of hilarity the adults tried to photograph us with their phones. They didn't even try to hide their actions. We quickly moved between and around cars to block their view of us. Fortunately, we were not followed. We'd planned to visit for the whole afternoon. But we left after only two hours – and a further three instances of unsolicited photographing.

On the fourth occasion, Sarah and I were walking over a

small footbridge in the gardens when a slightly built man walking towards us smirked and lifted his phone, pointing it directly at us from less than two metres away. We heard the click of the camera.

Before I could say anything, Sarah strode towards him. 'Excuse me. You just took a photo of us.'

He was clearly taken aback by being confronted. 'No, I didn't,' he said, blushing and looking down at the ground. In his discomfort, he forgot to hide the screen of his phone, which was now clearly visible.

Sarah pointed at the device. 'Yes, you did! It's really upsetting. We don't like it. It's not right. We didn't give our permission. Delete it immediately, please.'

The man appearing increasingly embarrassed – I suspect both at being found out in an obvious lie and at Sarah's assertiveness. He did exactly as she requested and muttered 'Sorry' – to which Sarah replied simply, 'Thank you.'

Walking away, I took a few cursory glances over my shoulder to make sure he wasn't continuing to photograph us, but he hurried away. Sarah was walking so briskly I had to run to catch up.

We weren't far from where we had left my husband looking after the puppies and our belongings. When we reached him, my first words to Sarah were, 'I'm immensely proud of the way you handled that. You were absolutely right, and you spoke to him appropriately. Well done. But you need to be careful if you are by yourself.'

I didn't say more, because Sarah had tears in her eyes. 'I just want to get out of here. I want to go home ,' she said.

We packed up our belongings, gathered the puppies and left.

This incident was bittersweet. Bitter, because Sarah was deeply distressed and we were denied the enjoyment of a simple afternoon outing, which made me incredibly angry. But simultaneously sweet, because I saw that my child had the self-esteem and wherewithal not to tolerate bad behaviour and to demand the respect we all rightly deserve. I could quietly reassure myself: 'She's got this!'

*

Sarah is now a young woman. She is a vet nurse, enjoys a social life with friends and family and is the proud parent of a furbaby, a mini-Australian shepherd. Sarah has lived all her life using step stools to reach things, needing alterations to her clothes, driving with modifications to her car and sometimes just having to accept that there are some things we simply can't do. She knows practical alterations will always be a part of her life because of her dwarfism – and that she will also have to manage careless, thoughtless and ill-mannered behaviour from others. She talks of one day having children herself. Then I will be called 'Nanny' – as Mum was called by my nieces and nephews. I am confident that should the time come when my daughter becomes a parent, she will reassure herself: 'I've got this!'

* * *

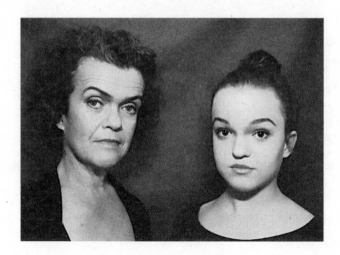

Debra Keenahan is a visual artist, psychologist, academic and author. Her work focusses upon the personal and social impacts of disability. Having achondroplasia dwarfism, she brings her individual insight to understanding of the dynamics of interpersonal interactions and social structures that include/exclude the visibly different from equitable social relations.

Kristen Witucki

from an interview with Eliza Hull

I've always been a dreamer. As a child, I remember having visions of one day having kids. I'd play with my dolls and make up stories. I was born blind, so growing up I noticed that other girls my age were encouraged to babysit, but I was never given that opportunity, except maybe when I looked after my younger brother. I didn't have much experience looking after kids until I was in college, studying to become a teacher.

During this time, I began dating. I remember one potential partner saying he liked me a lot but didn't actually want to get together, because I had a disability. He felt he would have to make too many allowances for it. So that made me worry whether I would ever find the right person.

Luckily, at age twenty-six, I met James and fell in love. He is blind also. I told him early on that I wanted to have children. He is older than I am and already had kids from a previous relationship. He was still very supportive of us starting a family together and wanted to make it a reality.

I remember feeling quite alone, though, in my decision to be a parent. I didn't know any other parents with disabilities. I didn't have anyone I could ask about having children other than James. But I still chose to take the leap.

The pregnancy itself went relatively well. One thing I noticed was the lack of excitement from others, especially strangers on the street. In the past, I noticed that random people would gush over other people's pregnancies, even if they didn't know them. When I was pregnant, I met only one such person who said they were excited for me. It's not like I wanted strangers to come up to me, but I guess I was seeking a stamp of approval from society for choosing motherhood.

During my twenty-week ultrasound, the baby was thought to have a mark on its heart which had a weak correlation to the possibility of Down's syndrome. The doctor recommended that I go to the hospital for a second opinion, so I went to the antenatal testing centre. Before he even got a good look at the baby's heart, one of the doctors there said, 'Oh, well, you know, if he has a heart condition, and because you have a disability, you should really consider terminating this pregnancy.' And I said, 'Isn't this a Catholic hospital? Aren't you supposed to not say that?' 'Oh, well, yeah,' he replied. 'But we would find where you could do it.'

To be honest, I started to believe the doctor. I started asking myself whether I should have this child. 'Can I do this?' And then I oscillated back to 'Why would he say that?' It surprised me how willing I was to give up on having a baby because of his judgement. In the end, the mark on its heart was a false alarm.

Before the baby was born, I went on a tour of the hospital and met several nurses. I alerted them to my existence and informed them that I was blind and would be giving birth there. Unfortunately, when my baby decided to arrive, none of the same staff were working. Babies don't arrive on people's shifts. The communication was very poor, because nobody knew I was coming. At times I felt like hospital staff didn't know how to speak and interact with me.

After a quick delivery, my gorgeous son Langston was born. Throughout my hospital stay with him, I was worried that somebody was going to take him away. I had read so many stories about it happening. So, in addition to all the normal first-time mother fears was the fear that if I did anything wrong, the hospital would take the baby. I was pretty much a wreck through that whole experience. As a person with a disability, perhaps I should have been more forceful about how I wanted to parent. But I took the opposite tack. I kept myself surrounded by people who loved me, and I loved, and I think the hospital just had this feeling that I live with these people all the time and that I had support networks in place. So, luckily, they left me alone.

Initially we took Langston home, but then he was tested for bilirubin levels, and they were high, so he had to go back into the hospital for a couple of days without me. I was very scared to leave him there, worried that this was going to be their chance to take him from my care. But once I figured out that the nurses were just interested in making sure he was getting better, I felt calmer. At the time, I was pumping breast milk and taking it in for him. It also was positive in that it gave me a chance to recoup

171

and recover for a couple of days, although I did miss him. When he came home for the second and final time, he was fine, which was a relief. My mom stayed with us for a couple more days to support our transition. I remember when she went home, I was at a loss. What were we going to do? Those first few months were monotonous and repetitive. Apart from occasional visits from friends, the days were very long and were just feed, change, sleep, repeat. I felt very isolated at times.

Since our first child, my partner and I have had two more kids, a boy named Noor and a girl named Karuna. For those births, I decided I was done with the hospital. I was very lucky to have home births instead, with certified nurse midwives who I knew and trusted, because I saw them throughout the whole pregnancy. There was never the question: can you take care of this baby? It was just so much more relaxing. I highly recommend it to anyone with a disability who's relatively low risk. For us, if anything went wrong, there were two hospitals within one or two miles from our house. So, we felt it was as safe as possible.

When the kids were babies, we had to learn ways to adapt. For instance, when they were sick, we had to find a dropper that was the same size as the dose of medicine needed. Then there were the talking thermometers. The ones I have used have been amazingly inaccurate, so I've mostly taken temperatures by touch. We read to the kids in braille and used a pram that is like a wagon. Conventional baby strollers are pushed at the front, and we can't use them because we use canes. So instead, we would pull the stroller behind us. Nappy changes weren't too hard. I had a friend, who, before they were born, simulated what cleaning poop out of a diaper would be like by putting mustard into her elbow crease. It was my way of learning how to change them.

You lose a lot of sleep taking care of babies, but they're also very tactile and audible little creatures. They make noise when they need help, and they don't move when you put them down. In some ways, they're not as hard as toddlers, who are always moving and who want a thousand things they can't say.

As my kids have started to grow up, I felt incredibly lucky, because I knew that if my two sons were quiet then something was going on, and I better check on them. They are very noisy, so it helped me a lot.

If we go out together to a park, I always check in with them to make sure I hear them. I also used to get them to wear these cute shoes which had squeakers inserted into them, so we could hear where they were running. I also used to use one of those leash backpacks, where the backpack is on the child and there's a band around my wrist. This helped when they didn't want to hold my hand.

Other times I would take a friend and they helped me by seeing where they were. I've had a lot of assistance in public places, especially when they were little. But at home, it's easy to set things up so that I always know where they are.

I am not sure exactly when the kids realised that we were both blind. I think they understood it in phases. From a very early age, all of them could communicate with me through touch and through sound and knew that they needed to do that. I remember a moment when my first baby was about a month old, I was getting those weekly emails tracking the baby's development. And one of the emails said all your hard work and sleep deprivation will soon be rewarded by your baby's first smile. And I remember feeling really depressed, because I was missing one of the most important milestones. I also worried my baby would smile at me and I would not smile back. And I was anxious I was ruining him. When he was two and a half months old, though, I remember singing him a song. He started to sort of sing with me in baby talk. And that really helped me to understand that our connection was unique and profound, and that even though I had missed some smiles, it was fine. We were fine. In a sense I feel like, even as babies, my kids knew that I couldn't see, they knew that they had to communicate differently with us. As they got older and were able to talk, they had the language to know we were blind. But my three-year-old still thinks if I open my eyes, maybe I will be able to see. I think she will figure out soon enough that won't work; she doesn't believe us yet. The other day she said, 'Mum, just open your eyes.'

The understanding of all three of my kids is always evolving. My two boys, who are now eleven and six, wish that we could see because they know what seeing is like. They haven't fully comprehended that because I was born blind, I don't need to see. Whenever my son has felt bad for me that I can't see, I say maybe I don't see the colours that you are, but I know you much, much better than most people who can see. Because I'm your mother. And right now, I probably know you better than anyone knows you.

Sometimes the boys try and get away with doing things like

making silly gestures. I say to them half joking but half seriously that if you lie to a blind person, then it's bad karma. I don't think they get away with too much.

Now as a family we go to parks with friends, or relatives, or sometimes I just go with them, we're lucky to have some great parks nearby where they can play, and sometimes my eleven-year-old can now look out for his siblings as well. Sometimes we will take the train into New York together and meet our friends there. It's always an adventure.

At the train station, I have heard people yell out to my kids to take care of your mom. My style is to hold in my anger, but sometimes I do wonder if I should say something. The truth is, if my kid was the one in charge, we would be dead. But I don't say that, because the kids do sometimes help. I don't want to dismiss their efforts. For instance, they may have read a sign for me that day or done something small that was helpful.

The kids don't fully understand yet about people's misconceptions about disability. They don't realise that people with disability have had to struggle to even get to this point, and how many barriers people with disability still must face in wider society. My kids are also biracial. I'm a white, European American and my husband is African American. I think they have much more consciousness about race and racism, especially my oldest son.

We've been lucky, though, overall, in our community. The kids have wonderful schoolteachers, who have been incredibly understanding. The other parents have been nice and helpful. We live in a beautiful little community, where it's easy to walk around. We're lucky in that way because we don't drive. We try to limit how much we seek support from the wider school community. If the weather is bad, sometimes we do need to ask for a ride, or if one of the kids is invited to a party and it's not within walking distance, then sometimes we'll reach out to see if they can get transportation. But besides that, I try not to bother people too much.

Parents have also been great at trusting us. I am still surprised when parents are comfortable with dropping their kids over.

If I was to give advice to any blind people contemplating starting a family, I would suggest trying to find other blind parents to connect with. Learn from their stories and ask lots of questions. I remember even when I had two children, I was comfortable with the more basic parenting, but I still wasn't sure about having a third child. I connected with a blind mother who had three children and just talked to her about some of the joys and challenges. And that was so helpful. I think if you feel that you are ready and willing and able to take care of a child, and have the love and the patience to do it, then don't let anyone stop you.

The best thing about parenting is getting really acquainted with people who're such completely different individuals from you. They're not going to grow up to be like you; they are their own people. Once you embrace that, it can be really liberating and exciting just to know you're having a role in shaping such unique human beings. My eldest child is really interested in science, especially animals, whereas I don't like hanging out with animals that much, so I feel a new appreciation for a perspective like his and try to support his interest, even though it's not one I share. My middle child is so social and extroverted. And his dad and I are both introverted, as is his brother and sister. I know he was born in my house, so there is no mistaking he is my baby. He really is so unique, and so wonderfully adventurous. So that's a lot of fun. I get to become friends with them and be their guardian. There's no other experience like it.

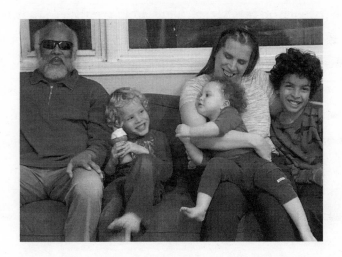

Kristen Witucki has been totally blind since birth. She was raised in New Jersey and earned a BA in English from Vassar College in 2004, with a minor in German and certification to teach students in grades 7–12. She followed it with three master's degrees: an MA in teaching gifted students, from Teachers College, Columbia University; an MFA in the creative writing of fiction, from Sarah Lawrence College; and an EdM in teaching students who are blind or visually impaired, from Dominican College. While in school, she earned her living at

Learning Ally, where she helped people with visual impairments, dyslexia and other disabilities to access technology related to reading audiobooks.

Kristen has completed two works of fiction: *The Transcriber*, a shorter book for adolescent emerging readers that is part of GemmaMedia's Open Door series, and *Outside Myself*, a novel. Her nonfiction has appeared in *The Huffington Post*, the Momoir Project, *Literary Mama* and *Brain, Child*.

Kristen is a teacher of blind and low-vision students for Vistas Education Partners, and a content writer for Tamman Inc. She has also served as a mentor for college students who are blind and, more recently, has mentored writers for the Association of Writers and Writing Programs. She lives in New Jersey with her husband and children.

Jacinta Parsons

When they held him up in the light, he looked otherworldly. We have a photo of him in that moment. It looks as if he has descended from heaven. He is being held aloft, all bloated grey flesh and blood smeared across his tiny body, against the harshness of the metal operating theatre, a golden light – fit for a king – streaming across him, like he was a prize we had won. Here he was, our beautiful child, born of our bodies.

I often look at that photo and wish that more of life could be like this. That we could press pause and hold a moment. Stay there, in stillness. How lovely it would be to have all movement and sound cease and for us to sink inside these perfect formations in time.

It should feel like that any time a child arrives on earth. A miracle. A child should always be bathed in perfect light, held up like the prize they are. But often everyday trauma bangs up against the miraculous, making it hard to see clearly.

Just on the other side of the photo, I'm there. Panicked, shivering, and sweating with the white heat of fear cursing through my blood. What the photo doesn't show is that he emerged from an imperfect, unhealthy body. Sickness had spewed him out just in the nick of time, when we worried he might not be safe. Months earlier, I had turned yellow and since then I had been visiting the hospital nearly every day to be hooked up to heart monitors and to test my blood, to make sure he was still alive.

The surgeon peered over the curtain between my head and a knife that was trained on my abdomen. 'No more children for you. You're lucky. We just missed cutting your bowel.'

'Thanks,' I whispered back, shocked that he had chosen this moment to tell me. But I didn't want to cause a fuss. My body was still open and all I wanted was for him to finish the unbearable tugging and stitching going on. My body had been wound up so tight, with such enormous fear, that every tiny sensation – even through the epidural – felt like a razor blade.

They put my baby on my chest, just like I'd seen in the birthing literature. But panic hit me, and I felt sick. The enormous chasm I felt between us : that isn't what they tell you you'll feel. I didn't know how I would ever make it across to him. I wanted to be different. I wanted to crawl out of my skin and escape. I wanted him to be held by someone who could love him well in that first moment of his life. The terror of bringing this life to earth had completely worn me out; I was see-through.

This was the second time I had been here, at the crossroads of life and death. The thinnest of membranes between the worlds. Giving birth.

*

The first hurdle that you face as a parent with a disability or chronic illness is actually becoming one. My body had become so unreliable that it frightened me. And the idea of bringing a life through this skin and bones that had caused so much pain felt almost too much to bear.

I had slowly become accustomed to the danger of my sick body – the pain, the fragility, the exposure to the reality of my mortality through its capacity for malfunction. I had been diagnosed with Crohn's disease and had developed fistulas throughout my perianal area and vagina and now had an ileostomy bag.

The idea that this body might be responsible for producing another life was overwhelming. I would become breathless at the hugeness of the task. The idea of attempting to house a child in this hostile body brought me such grief. What if my body couldn't become pregnant? And worse still, what if it could become pregnant but could not stay well enough to keep a child safe? I felt grief for my old life, the one I'd taken for granted before illness, when I had been innocent to the reality of how fragile we all really are.

The grief was also about all the other dreams that I was destroying. My partner's, his family's, my family's, and those of the little girl who had thought she would one day be a mum. It was all my fault.

The guilt and grief intermingled like a dirty puddle – it was difficult to see them separately. I felt like I was drowning in the disappointment of my failed body. Not only had I become difficult to live with because my needs had drastically changed, but the magic ability I had been promised was within my power as a woman – to carry a new life – was now looking out of reach.

When I was first diagnosed with Crohn's disease, the first question I asked the young doctor who diagnosed me was about my fertility. 'Well, there's no real reason why not,' he answered at the time. But what he failed to tell me was that chronic diseases have a life of their own. They will mutate in various wild and wonderful ways. What he should have said was that he couldn't tell me what might happen for me. Disease would make prediction impossible.

*

The conception of our first child was akin to magic. We had been trying for years to fall pregnant and had realised that with me as sick as I was it would be very unlikely. We had started the process of wondering what it would be like to be childless. Or might we try for a different course? Adoption? Foster care?

But somehow, in the middle of one of my sickest periods, when I was on a cocktail of drugs, we found out that a tiny life had found her way to us. The initial unbridled joy, turned into fear, as we crept our way towards hoping we could give birth to a child without my disease causing complications. 'Shhh,' I remember thinking, 'don't make too much noise. We don't want anyone to notice that we've won a prize.' I was so frightened that somehow it would be taken away from us.

During the almost nine months I was pregnant that first time, it felt like we were tiptoeing through every day, not quite daring to feel the excitement of her possibility.

I had a specialist obstetrician at the hospital and support from my bowel surgeons, but she decided she wanted to arrive early – on a long weekend when none of the doctors who had been preparing for this birth were available.

It all happened so quickly. I found myself in an operating theatre with an anaesthetist who decided I should be put under a general anaesthetic to give birth. As I went to sleep, surrounded by strangers, I remember begging everyone in the room to do their best job. As if my pleas might make it more likely for them to care if we lived or died. It was so strange to leave the conscious world knowing that I would wake to an outcome but that I would have no control over what happened in the interim.

The anaesthetist promised to write on my hand what had happened. Whether it was a boy or a girl, and what time they had arrived. As soon as I woke, I held my shaking hand up so that I could read the words through my groggy eyes : '8.49 pm. girl.'

And with that, I was undone. I had held myself together so tightly through the entire journey. That she had arrived without me, but safely, was almost too much. We had done it. We had won the golden prize. But it had also broken something inside me that I'm not sure I have yet put back together.

After we brought her home, I didn't think I could ever have another child. It frightened me too much. I didn't feel free with my love anymore. It felt too dangerous to love when I had felt so viscerally an imminent potential loss.

*

When I became pregnant for a second time, eight years after the first, I was still experiencing a type of trauma from that first birth. In the months leading up to my son's birth, I had become unwell with a liver condition and was in and out of hospital daily.

Having had so much go wrong with my health up until that point, I feared the inevitability of this second birth not going to plan. In a strange way, the liver diagnosis gave me some relief. Finally knowing the thing that had gone wrong meant I could breathe out. I had found out exactly what it was that I was up against this time.

Before they laid him on my chest in that first moment of his life, I think I had tried hard to leave my body. The pain felt too much. Illness and danger had finally become too heavy and impenetrable. The responsibility of bearing our children had been too much for this broken form to be trusted with.

So when at last he arrived, I found it difficult to understand that we were both safe. I had to remind myself that he was okay and it was safe now to let my guard down. But it took me a long time. I cried for weeks after his birth.

For me, parenting has made me feel raw about my illness. It has exposed the deepest fears I have, ones that have usually been kept down below the surface. Parenting has meant they have risen inside me so I can't ignore them.

My entire family have had to adjust to me parenting with chronic illness. But while there has been enormous pain, it has also been one of the greatest tools I have in my parenting armoury.

In the early years of parenting our first child, I distinctly remember her disappointment in me. Often I was too tired to play. Or I just couldn't sit or stand too long without needing to rest. I would make excuses for why I wanted to play a game that meant I had to lie on the couch. Or sometimes I would ask her to play with me from my bed.

She approached me, one afternoon, very cross. She was still little, but it was clear to her that I could be doing much more to get better. I was lying in bed and she came up close to my face and started pulling on my arm.

'Can you get up?' she demanded.

'Sorry, babe, I'm not feeling well. Maybe in a minute,' I begged.

She continued to pull on my arm as her anger began to rise. 'Mum, get up!' she yelled. 'Why don't you go to a doctor to get better?' she cried at me. 'Why don't you just take some medicine?' She stormed out of the room, angry that nothing she could do could make me move. And I lay there wondering if she was right. Perhaps I hadn't been doing everything I should have been doing. Perhaps it was my fault that I was lying around. *Am I lazy?* I wondered.

Many parents harbour guilt for their parenting. A sense that you will be responsible for a child who has suffered your bad decisions . Most parents, especially when they start out, wonder if they should be giving more, working less, riding more bikes, making more playdough. But having illness compounds those fears. Every anxiety is magnified because you are not the parent you perhaps imagined you might have been. You are possibly not the parent you wish you could be. You're tired and in pain and your fuse is shorter than it should be. And when they look at you the way my daughter did that day, there is a big part of you that believes they are right. You have let them down.

It seemed so hard to explain to a child that I wasn't able to get better. At least not with all the medicine I had taken and all the surgery I had had so far. How do you explain to a child that sometimes illness can never leave you? That it can become part of who you are?

I searched the internet for an answer. But I found no resources to help me explain what it's like to have a parent with a chronic illness. There were plenty of materials on cancer and how to explain terminal illness, but nothing to help me find the words to explain to her that I was sick and that the sickness was going to be how we lived.

I realised that the management of my illness had been hidden from her. While she had seen me in hospital, it hadn't made much sense. She didn't understand that I was always seeing a doctor and always working on how to live with this illness. She couldn't imagine the world that I lived in, because she hadn't really seen it.

I decided to tell her all about the doctors who cared for me. I told her their names and what they looked like. I told her details about where they worked and which hospital I travelled to, to see them. I explained what the rooms looked like, and all the things that I did when I was there. Blood tests, sometimes scans, weighing. I told her they were kind and they looked after me really well. Even though I was tired and sore, being sick was part of who I was and that was okay.

As the years went on and she grew, we started to have conversations about what illness has taught me and continues to teach me. How it showed me I was strong. How it opened up the world for me in ways I wouldn't have understood without it. And I explained that I wouldn't choose not to have this illness if I had the option. It is now who I am.

We know as a family that we are perfect in our imperfections and that there is no such thing as normal. I have been open with them both, through the years of our lives together, that some of this has been hard. I have made sure that I haven't shielded this from them because what they always see is that eventually I get up again. Falling down doesn't have to be frightening when you know deep down that you'll eventually find a way to get up.

And we have learnt that we can never judge any moment — we have no idea what will come from the lives we are asked to lead. There are jewels hidden in the most unlikely places.

I have worked hard to shake the internal voice that tells me that my illness has made me less than. Less than the parent that I might have been.

My parenting was cast in the fire of illness. It is impossible to know me as a woman or a mum without understanding me as having illness. It is the frame for everything I know, and everything I would love them to one day understand.

I see my illness for all the richness it has afforded our family. A depth of empathy. An understanding of how we need to be flexible in the face of change. To make decisions around our challenges, even if they're only small choices. To have patience. To be kind.

My children have also learnt that our bodies can let us down. But that our bodies are not the totality of who we are. And we're not to be afraid of where it will take each of us. We never know where the journey might lead.

My youngest child announces proudly to anyone who will listen, 'My mum has chronic illness, you know.' As if it's something we have won. A prize. And in many ways, I think he's right.

When I look at that photo of the moment he was born, I remember there is another side to it. And that I live on that other side. But what I know now is that the story didn't end in that moment. Not for either of us. It was only the beginning of something rich and hard and beautiful and wild. And the prize was the rest of it: every moment of our lives that has followed since. Not perfect, but life.

* * *

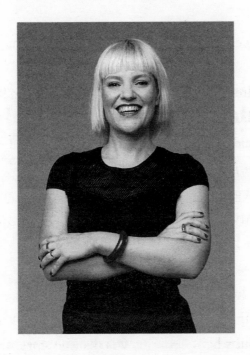

Jacinta Parsons is a broadcaster, radio maker, writer, public speaker and author of the memoir *Unseen: The Secret Life of Chronic Illness*. She currently hosts *Afternoons* on ABC Melbourne, delivering a popular mix of art, culture and ideas.

Jaclyn and Garry Lynch

from an interview with Eliza Hull

Garry and I met in October 2009, at a disability enterprise in the eastern suburbs of Melbourne. Garry has Asperger's syndrome, which was diagnosed at the age of seven when he started school. He had a Teacher's Aid, which made him feel inadequate and different. As an adult, his disability affects him in the way he feels: he is often overloaded and tired, especially after a long day at work.

I was born with a brain tumour, which caused severe epilepsy. For the first two years of my life I wouldn't stop crying. Mum knew that something wasn't right. She kept going to doctors, saying, 'There is something wrong with my baby', but they kept sending her away saying I was fine, there was nothing to worry about. I can't imagine what that would have been like for Mum, nobody listening to her.

When I was three, I had my first epileptic seizure. From then on, I was having fits every hour. When I was fifteen, the doctors decided to operate and remove a tumour they found with an MRI scan. After the operation, the seizures stopped, but unfortunately the tumour grew back, so I had to have surgery again. Throughout my childhood I continued to have seizures, which led to me falling behind in my learning. For this reason, I now have an intellectual disability. I used to have very large seizures. I would shake and collapse on the floor, and then I would fall asleep for an hour or two, wake up and then have another kind of seizure where I would just stop and stare.

Now, as an adult, I have times when I forget things for a bit. I also have some memory loss. There are some things I find hard to learn, but there are other areas where I am very capable.

When Garry and I first met, we instantly connected. We have a lot in common but we are also opposites in many ways, I love to have conversations and he likes to listen. Eleven years later, here we are, still in love. Very early on, I remember telling him I was keen to have children. He was always a little more uncertain and apprehensive, but quickly he came around, and together we decided we would start a family.

For two years we tried for a baby, but we had no luck conceiving. A doctor recommended that I be placed on hormone tablets to help, and at last I finally fell pregnant. Garry was both nervous and happy – he had very mixed feelings, whereas I felt pure excitement.

Unfortunately, this excitement was short-lived as I had a miscarriage. During this time, Garry was diagnosed with Stage 2 Hodgkin's lymphoma. We were both very scared and knew we needed to move quickly, so we had his sperm frozen. We didn't want to take any chances, and his sperm might be affected by the cancer treatment. Two weeks later we were placed on the emergency list and given the chance to conceive again through the use of artificial insemination. Luckily this pregnancy was successful. As it progressed, we both became more and more excited. It began feeling like a reality, like we were actually going to have a family.

During the pregnancy Garry was vomiting because of his cancer treatment, and I was vomiting because I was pregnant: we were both so sick! Funnily, though, this actually brought us closer together because we needed to rely on each other for support.

Garry was very nervous and uncertain throughout the nine months of pregnancy, hoping it would all work out. I was fortunate because I had a lot of experience with kids. My sisters got me to look after their children when they were little, so I had had a lot of practice. I remember watching my mum and how she looked after my nieces and nephews. I learnt a lot from her, and then she would let me look after them with her assistance so I could take it all in. When my mum and dad went away on a holiday around Australia, my sister Becky asked if I could help her look after her kids. I changed nappies and fed the baby while my sister was at work. I fell in love with the experience and that was when I knew that having my own children was something I wanted in my life. I knew I'd be a good, caring mother.

After nine long months (I say long because I was nauseous the whole time), I finally gave birth to our adorable little boy Riley. I had wanted a natural birth, but his umbilical cord was wrapping around him during the labour and the doctors rushed me off to have a caesarean. Garry cut the umbilical cord. I remember saying to the doctor, 'As soon as you take out the baby, can you tell me the time?' It ended up being 2:30 pm on the dot. I am not sure why I wanted to know the exact time of birth; it was just something I'd been looking forward to hearing. Holding my beautiful baby boy was a better feeling than I could ever have imagined. You should have seen Garry! He was walking up and down the hospital corridors saying, 'Look at my baby, everyone!' Right from the beginning he was such a proud father. It was one of the best days of his life; actually, it was the best thing that ever happened to both of us, nothing else would ever compare.

While we were riding the high of having our first baby, things started to unravel. During those first few days, when I reached out for support within the hospital I was met with discrimination and judgement. For parents with intellectual disability in Australia, the system is not in your favour. It's almost like people are waiting to catch you out, to make you look like you're doing something wrong, to prove that you're unable to take care of your child.

I was advised that we should go to a parenting program, where we would need to stay for a week to help with the sleeping and feeding routine. My mum also suggested it might be a good idea, so we agreed to give it a go. We had only been there for two days before Child Protection was called. When the staff in the parenting program realised I was epileptic, they thought I was having a fit while holding Riley. In fact, I was having an anxiety attack because my hormones were shifting. Like a lot of new mothers, I was overwhelmed and needed some support.

Right from the beginning, we did not feel safe at the parenting centre: instead, we felt like we were constantly being monitored. They tried to say that we had given Riley a bottle that was too hot – but we hadn't. Garry had made up a bottle of formula and had forgotten to test the temperature himself. But I tested the temperature before I gave it to Riley and asked Garry to go and cool it down. The lady at the parenting centre watched this all take place, she knew this is how it happened, yet she decided to use the situation to frame us as incapable to parent. We felt we had been set up.

My mum came in that day to have a look at the place and see how we were going. As she arrived, we were already being called into a separate room to have a meeting with Child Protection. During these initial meetings they didn't give us any support people or any of the documentation in Plain English. Nothing was accessible. They told me they thought I was a danger to my child, but I tried to tell them that I knew I hadn't had a seizure, it was anxiety caused by the stress.

When my mother walked into the meeting, they tried to put Riley into her arms. Mum was quick to say, 'No, he needs to stay with his mother.' Mum knows me better than anybody else; she knows how competent I am, and she knew how capable I was of looking after my baby.

The Department of Health and Human Services kept pushing me to put Riley on the bottle; I was so upset because I wanted to continue to breastfeed him. He was starting to lose weight, though, so they pressured me to stop. In the end we found out he had a tongue-tie and that was why he was losing weight. If a maternal health nurse had given me support instead of continually dismissing me, we could have realised that together. Then, as with many babies who have a tongue-tie, it could have been resolved and I could have breastfed my child.

After many meetings with Child Protection, it was agreed that Riley could stay in my care if my mother lived with us at our house. They said my mother would have to live with me until Riley was at least one year old. Mum got very upset and said, 'I can't do that. I am married and have a husband to be with. I can't sleep on their couch forever.' In the end, Riley and I moved in with Mum. At first Garry had to stay behind because his work was too far away from where Mum lived. It was hard being separated from him. Luckily, he found another job that was nearby, so he moved in with Mum as well. We stayed there for six months, until my sister and brother took over and we got a house to share with them, so I could still be with my son.

Throughout this time, we were so scared that Child Protection was going to separate us from our son. It was just this constant feeling of being watched, that any day our baby could be taken away. It was so distressing.

Child Protection really wanted Riley out of our lives; the lady who was our contact person seemed to want us to fail. She would try to manipulate me when she did her weekly home visits; often it felt like she was trying to push me to make a mistake. I was told that we wouldn't be able to have Riley in our care without family support in our house until he went to school. At this stage I sought advice from a disability advocacy organisation, VALID. They were incredible at outlining what my rights were as a parent with intellectual disability. They taught me ways to demonstrate competency to Child Protection by documenting evidence such as tabling times and dates of feeds and taking photos and video footage of washing Riley and preparing formula so we could demonstrate our parenting skills and abilities. I was also lucky that we had family who recommended a good lawyer, who represented us when the Department of Health and Human Services took us to court. In the trial, Child Protection tried to twist things to make us look bad. It was so debilitating and disempowering. Fortunately, though, we won. They didn't have any proof of our incapacity to parent, and we were able to show how capable and committed we were to our son. As the court case concluded, the judge commended me and apologised that I had to go through such a traumatic experience.

Riley is now four years old. He is a beautiful, caring little boy. Child Protection leaves us alone now. Really, they should never have been called; they should never have forced me to live with my mother or my siblings. But the staff at the parenting centre get scared as soon as they have parents with disabilities. To me, it's obvious they don't have the appropriate training and experience with parents with disability. Because it's a centre for everyone: for people with disability and non-disabled people. It felt like as soon as they had someone with a disability in their centre they rang Child Protection. It felt like blatant discrimination. They were so quick to judge, without waiting to see what we were capable of or offering any support.

In retrospect, I wish I hadn't listened to the hospital staff when they suggested we go there. It was sold to me as a place where we would be supported, where we could learn, but they just scrutinised us – tested us and made us feel like we were incompetent.

Luckily, we feel safe now. Now that we've proved it in court, I don't think they would come for us if we had another child, because they know now that I am a great parent, we both are.

Life is now calm. Garry works and I am a stay-at-home mother. Riley goes to kinder three days a week. He is a gorgeous, loving little boy; he makes us both so happy. He constantly gives us hugs and kisses. I don't think he realises that we both have a disability. He definitely knows the word 'disabled', though, and often will check in with us to see how we are. He really is a good kid. We talk about disability in the home, because we are both proud of our disabilities. He doesn't really understand yet that we both have a disability, but when he grows up we will teach him that it's not a negative thing, and that it's important to treat everyone the same way. Life has been a lot smoother since we are out of the Child Protection system. We feel accepted within our community. The other parents at Riley's kindergarten include us whenever possible.

As a family, we love to watch movies together. We also go out shopping or spend quality time together going to the park. There are certain things that Riley relies on from each of us. For instance, I am not a great reader so that is something Garry takes over with. I also don't drive, but Garry does. I am good with assisting with the toilet, whereas Garry struggles with quick instructions. We help each other out and use our individual strengths to raise him well.

I feel like a very capable parent. We are lucky, as we have a lot of family support. My mum only lives down the road so if we ever need her, she's there. My dad is also close by, so if there is ever an emergency or anything we need he can be on my doorstep within minutes. It's wonderful for Riley to have his extended family in his life. He loves them and they adore playing with him and having fun.

I think often people are quick to judge. They think that if someone has an intellectual disability, we won't know how to do this or that. There are so many misconceptions about being a parent with intellectual disability. It's really wrong. I feel people need more education. It's been really hard to push up against. I am tired of having to prove to people that I can parent. What other parent has to do that?

I know I am a great mother, and Garry is a wonderful father. We can parent, we give it our all, and we love our little boy so much. The best thing about being a parent is being able to witness our son grow and develop and enjoy himself and have fun in life! Witnessing this makes it all worth it.

* * *

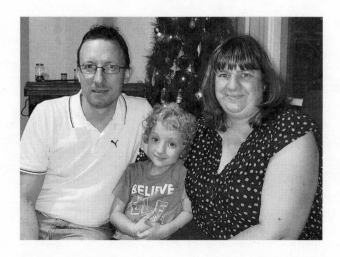

Jaclyn Lynch is a proud parent with intellectual disability. **Garry Lynch** has autism spectrum disorder (ASD). They both work with Legal Aid's Independent Family Advocacy Service and self-advocacy group Positive Powerful Parents.

Brent Phillips

from an interview with Eliza Hull

Being Deaf has never felt different to me: it is what I've always known. My parents and grandparents are also Deaf, so I grew up within Deaf culture. It was normalised and engrained in me. As a child, I saw that Deaf people could be wonderful parents – and because I had my own Deaf parents as role models, I was confident I could be a great parent myself.

I met my partner, Mel, in 2006 and fell in love at first sight. Mel is also Deaf, as are her parents, so together we have Deafness in our genetics. It's something we are both deeply proud of.

Seven years later, in 2013, our daughter Taylor was born. The first couple of days with her were bliss. We were elated. She was everything we could ever have imagined and more.

When Taylor was just three days old, a nurse came buzzing into our hospital room to do the hearing screening test, an initiative funded by the government where every newborn is screened for hearing loss. We weren't given the opportunity to have an interpreter present, so we had to rely on lip reading. I vividly remember watching the nurse speak after completing the test on Taylor. She put out her hand to shake mine and said excitedly, 'Congratulations!'

Mel and I looked at each other, puzzled. What did she mean? Congratulations because she's like us? She's Deaf? Or congratulations, your daughter has passed the test and can hear? We were confused, but we quickly realised she was congratulating us that our daughter could hear. Our lack of enthusiasm must have surprised her. We didn't care at all if our daughter was hearing or not; to us, this wasn't a matter of passing or failing. She was perfect either way.

I started to imagine what the nurse would say to parents whose babies 'failed' the test. She'd probably say 'I'm sorry' and feel pity for them. This thought made me so sad. I wish that nurses would support parents in that moment and educate them about Deaf culture and the amazing community that exists out there. The cultural and linguistic perspective on deafness is so different to the way it is viewed in the medical model. But the medical world has so much power; deafness is still often seen as a deficit. And if this is how a hearing parent is introduced to the idea of deafness, they may have no idea what a positive world their child can be part of.

Thankfully, the next day, we drove home from the hospital with Taylor in the backseat. I was so cautious with our new precious cargo on board. In our Melbourne apartment – our own little bubble – we were all set up with everything we needed. We had what is called a baby cry alarm to alert us in the night when Taylor would make a noise or cry. The noise receptor was placed near her cot and we had a pager we could carry when we were in the lounge room or our bedroom. As soon as she made a noise, it would vibrate and flash to alert us.

From day one we signed to Taylor in Auslan. We would sign 'milk', 'sleep', 'mummy' and 'daddy'. She couldn't comprehend it for a while of course, but we just kept going. After a few months she started to respond by mimicking, and by nine months she was signing words and communicating freely with us.

Two years later, my son Nate was born. He is also hearing. He too was signing in Auslan by nine months. I am very proud that both our kids learnt Auslan as their first, native language.

Often people ask me, 'How did the children learn to speak?' We guess they must have picked up their English and spoken language from TV and from hearing family members – aunties, uncles and cousins – speaking. When they turned one, they began childcare a couple of days a week: that's where their spoken language really took off.

But we were never too concerned about how specifically they would pick up English; we knew they'd pick it up eventually. Our priority was for our home to be an Auslan environment, where we could all communicate in the same language.

For a long time, I don't think the children even noticed we were Deaf. Since their grandparents are also Deaf, it's something they have always grown up around. But at childcare they began to notice that other children communicated with their parents verbally. So perhaps it was then that they began to understand that we signed because we couldn't hear.

They would tap us on the shoulder and say, 'There's a dog

outside barking' or let us know that someone was at the door. We have visible alert systems for when someone comes to the door, but sometimes the children would let us know they heard a noise.

When Taylor was just three years old and Nate was a baby, we had a cry alarm set up in Nate's room but not in the laundry or some other spaces in the house. When Nate began crawling, he would move into these other rooms and occasionally he would cry out. Taylor would often say, 'Dad, Nate is in there' and point to where Nate was. It was just a natural part of them growing up that they understood their parents couldn't hear.

When the kids were young, before financial support from the National Disability Insurance Scheme (NDIS) was rolled out, we didn't have access to interpreters. When we attended birthday parties for hearing kids, we would feel extremely awkward. Mel and I would just stand there and try to gesture to people. We felt uneasy. The party was alive and we were trying to keep up. Often I would shadow Taylor, following her around just to keep myself busy. I'd throw a ball or join in a physical game with the kids to distract myself from communicating with the other parents. It could feel lonely at times.

When the NDIS was brought in, both Mel and I received funding packages. It meant we could finally book interpreters. This made a huge difference, because they could come along to the parties. It means we can now have in-depth conversations with the kids and their parents and not feel isolated. We bring an interpreter to the kids' sports matches too, so that we can communicate with the coach and other parents there. Everyone's become used to our interpreter coming along. Sometimes other parents ask us, 'How do you get an interpreter?' It gives me an opportunity to explain about the NDIS. Then they often ask more about our language. Sometimes they leave the conversation wanting to learn Auslan.

I'm not sure if Taylor or Nate had delays in speaking English. I don't think so. Certainly now, in primary school, they are fluent in both English and Auslan. We always read to them a lot from a young age. People often wonder how we go about doing that. The answer is we sign the stories to them in Auslan, but in English word order. Auslan has a completely different grammar, syntax and structure to English. But you can deliberately sign in English word order. Sometimes I use my voice to read to them, but I don't speak like a hearing person. I'm Deaf, and my voice reflects that.

One Saturday I took my son to Auskick. He was running around the oval and being a bit silly. So I called out to him, using my voice.

He quickly came over to me with a worried look on his face, and said, 'Do you know why that woman looked at you?'

I asked, 'Why, Nate?'

He replied, 'It's because you have a weird voice.'

I said, 'Well, yeah, Daddy does have a different voice. It's not like other people's voice. I can't hear myself speak. So I sound different.'

Our kids understand my voice because they're used to me; they have heard me every day of their lives. If I call out 'What do you want for dinner?', they understand what I'm saying and respond. But now that they are old enough to understand, I can explain that I sound different because I can't hear my voice and nobody's taught me how I should say certain words. Nate took this in his stride – he just said 'Okay' and ran off to keep playing.

The kids' teachers tell us their English is exceptional. When we started looking into schools for our children to go to, we did a lot of research. It was important to us to find a school that recognised and embraced the fact that we are a Deaf family and our children are bilingual. The school we ended up choosing had Italian as their second language at the time. After conversations with the principal, who was very supportive, they sent out a survey to the school community to nominate a language to replace Italian. Auslan was by far the most popular choice, so now they teach Auslan as the second language at the school. There are pros and cons to this. My kids are so fluent in both Auslan and English, they're often bored in their Auslan classes. Sometimes they even help teach the other kids. But one positive aspect is that it has helped us to integrate with the school community. Almost all the kids can sign now, or at least use the basic alphabet. So when they come over to our place, we can communicate with them. Some parents have even expressed interest in learning Auslan as well. That shows me that we have a very open-minded community and we are embraced and accepted. Our kids are proud of the fact they speak Auslan.

I've heard stories of kids who become embarrassed about using Auslan or who are teased in the schoolyard because their parents are Deaf. Luckily for our kids, because the other children and teachers use Auslan every day it is considered a normal part of school life. That's important for their self-esteem, their confidence and their pride in their native language, which we've instilled from early childhood.

We've always talked to our kids about how everyone is different. We explain that we are an example of that: because we can't hear, we use a visual language. We're lucky because we live in a very diverse area of Coburg; it's very multi cultural and progressive. Our kids have grown up seeing diversity as the norm, which is very different to my own childhood. When I was young, everyone around me was white and had a nuclear family, and gay people couldn't get married. I'm extremely pleased that my children are growing up in a world where diversity is embraced on multiple levels.

Nate is only six years old, and Taylor is just eight. Sometimes I wonder what will happen when they become teenagers. Will they become more self-conscious? That's why it's so important to invest in the relationships now with open communication.

When we are out in the local community, Taylor sometimes interprets for us without me asking her to. For instance, in the takeaway shop, when I go to write down my order, she will quickly interject, saying, 'I want to interpret for you, Dad,' without me prompting her. We've never forced our kids to interpret for us, but if they want to then we allow it. I'm very careful about it though, because I don't want to exploit their ability to hear and speak. I'm also very mindful to show them that Mum and Dad are independent – that we can function and communicate without relying on them.

As Deaf parents of two hearing children, we have provided them access to an entire other community and language and they love attending Deaf community events. They've got the best of both worlds: their local school community and the Deaf community.

For me, what was really important was instilling strong values and attitudes within our children. That growing up they would be allies of the Deaf community. They're proud of our family identity, and they can navigate both the Deaf world and the hearing world beautifully.

* * *

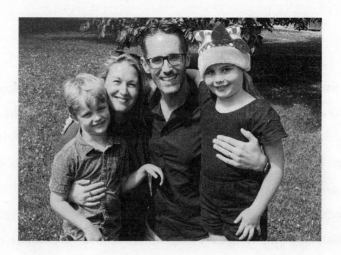

Brent Phillips is a third-generation Deaf person, married to a Deaf person and is the proud father of two children. Brent is currently Chief Impact Officer at Deaf Services and was Branch Manager – Assistive Technology & Employment Outcomes at the NDIA. He was formerly Chair of the Victorian Disability Advisory Council and Director – Language, Partnerships & Innovation at Expression Australia.

Mandy McCracken

It was one of the nurses who reminded me I should speak to my children. To be fair, I had a bit on my mind – I'd been in hospital for over two months. A streptococcal A infection had led to sepsis and to survive my hands and feet had just been amputated.

I was bloody lucky – and grateful – to be alive, but I hadn't expected to become disabled at thirty-nine. I'd never even met a single-leg amputee, let alone someone with both their hands and feet missing. *Was life like this still worth living?* The question bounced around in my head as I stared at the ceiling for hours on end. But I dare not say it aloud: like it or not, my new disability was something that my family and I were going to have to get used to.

The morning I was taken away in an ambulance, Samantha, our eldest daughter, had huddled in bed with her two little sisters, keeping them calm by reading stories. We should have been celebrating her ninth birthday that day – instead, Mummy went to hospital.

'I can help you,' the nurse suggested. 'I'll hold the phone to your ear and you could say good night to them. It will be easy.'

My husband Rod and I lived in Kilmore, a small town in regional Victoria, where I had a busy life as a stay-at-home mum of three. I volunteered at the kids' primary school and kinder, was on the local playground committee and headed the school's parents and friends committee. I did aerobics twice a week and played netball on Wednesday nights. We had even won two grand finals and I proudly displayed my first-ever trophies on the bookshelf at home, in all their shiny, plastic glory. My life looked just how I'd imagined it would . I was enjoying time with my daughters in the blissful first decade before they became teenagers and wanted me to leave them alone. I'd go back to work then, to help pay off the mortgage.

But now here I was, flat on my back in a hospital gown, bandaged from the shoulders down, with empty bed sheets where my feet should have been.

Although I appreciated the nurse reminding me of my parenting responsibilities, her comment prickled. Honestly, I was a little embarrassed that I'd forgotten about them. But with Rod doing a brilliant job of keeping them settled, my focus was simply on getting better.

I was on edge when, the next evening, the phone rang loudly on my bedside table and she dashed into my room to answer it. She lifted the receiver just moments too late.

'Argh, missed it, sorry ,' she said.

The scene repeated several times. A flurry of nurses came and went, running backwards and forwards from the nurse's station as my family tried to reach me. Hot and sweaty, the nurse finally said a brief hello before holding the phone to my ear.

'Hi, Mummy,' a tiny voice squeaked on the other end.

'Hello, gorgeous!' I beamed and instantly began to relax. 'It's so good to hear your voice. How was school today?' I was unsure which of my youngest two children I was talking to and hoped a few extra words might help me work it out. 'Good,' she answered.

'What did you learn about in class?'

'Not much.'

It was my middle daughter, Isobel. She was only seven and not the chattiest kid on the phone. I went on asking questions, trying my best to steer her away from one-word answers, without much success. Then I asked to speak to her younger sister.

'Hi, Mummy.' Tess, aged four, was slightly more open to a conversation, but only just. I tried to keep my voice light and engaging but the effort was rather exhausting in the circumstances.

The young nurse silently shifted on her feet. No doubt her arm was beginning to ache as she held the phone to my ear. The hospital ward was completely full and staff were always under the pump, so perhaps she was glad the kids weren't chattier.

I spoke briefly to Samantha before finally it was Rod's turn. 'Hi, babe. The girls are so excited to speak to you.'

'They don't have much to talk about,' I said sadly. I knew he could hear the disappointment in my voice. 'I've really let them down, haven't I?'

'Don't ever think that,' he replied. 'You know they love you and this is not your fault. Give it some time ... it will get easier.'

The next night my phone rang just as a nurse pushed through

the curtains. 'I'm right in the middle of a dressing change, can I prop the phone up and come back later?' she asked, looking flustered and blowing her fringe out of her eyes.

'Sure, take your time.'

Coming around my bed, she grabbed the phone and quickly held it to my ear before jamming a pillow at my shoulder.

'All set?'

I nodded and she left the room.

'Hello?'

'Hi, Mummy, it's Tess.'

'Tessy!' *God, she sounds so little.*

I asked about her day at kinder. We chatted about her teacher, what she'd had for lunch and the friends she played with. Then suddenly the phone slipped from my ear. I just managed to catch it with my chin.

'Honey, I'm dropping the phone. Can I say a quick hello to Isobel?'

Issy's voice squeaked on the line.

'Honey, I'm sorry but I'm dropping the phone.' Before she got a word in, the handset plummeted to the floor with a smash. I strained to call out to the phone beneath my bed. 'Issy! I'm so sorry but the phone is on the floor and I can't get it ... Just hang up and I'll speak to you tomorrow.'

An excruciating twenty minutes passed until the nurse finally returned.

'It's under the bed ,' I said flatly, staring out the window.

She picked up the phone and held it briefly to her ear. Nobody was there. Returning it to the cradle, she apologised in a faint voice and quickly left the room.

That night I cried waves of tears for my girls back home.

*

The following weekend Rod brought the three girls in to visit me. By now I'd been away from home for almost three months. Although Rod had explained to them everything that had happened, we knew their first visit would be difficult.

The curtain parted and three little faces slowly appeared.

'Hi, girls!' It was so good to see them – but they all looked completely terrified. They were dressed in their finest, their hair carefully brushed and plaited in a style I'd never seen before.

'Say hello to Mummy.' Rod gently pulled Isobel and Tess by their hands towards me.

Nine-year-old Samantha was the only one to move forward herself to stand by my bed. 'Hi.'

Spying a chair in the corner, Isobel and Tess quickly retreated there.

For five minutes or so we talked lightly about school and life at home – but I knew they were really waiting to see what had happened to their mum.

'Okay, come over here and have a look at my arms.'

Tess jumped up from the chair and stood rigid by my bed. Holding up a tiny pointed finger she gently pressed at my bandages.

'Don't hurt her,' said Samantha firmly, tugging Tess's hand away.

212

'It's okay, Sammy, it doesn't hurt.' In a calm voice, I explained what had happened. How the doctors had given me medicine to help me go to sleep and how, with a special knife, they had cut off my hands and feet. With Issy listening silently from the chair in the corner, Samantha and Tess asked all sorts of questions as they walked around my bed lifting the sheets to look at my legs. After ten minutes or so, they'd seen enough; their little faces relaxed, content that the situation was under control.

'Show Mummy what you've brought for her.' Rod held up a big bag and Samantha and Tess began unpacking their goodies. Isobel decided it was safe to join in and together the four of them filled my hospital room with handmade paintings and cards. They took it in turns to explain the pictures, and Rod stood on a chair and tacked their work to the walls. They finished by placing a teddy bear on a shelf near my bed.

Now my room was ablaze with colour and over the following months the girls added to it every week. As word got out among our community about what had happened to me, they brought in hundreds of cards and drawings from their classmates and other families back home.

Weeks went by, and I got used to my hospital bed being covered in tiny shoes and socks from Tess crawling in next to me. Being incredibly careful not to bump Mummy's sore arms or legs, Tess and Samantha often relaxed on the bed with their new mum.

Isobel was the last to climb up. She always began her visits sitting in the corner of the room. We didn't want to rush her: she was comfortable there. Finally, one day while the others were hanging paintings, she came and stood by my bed and gently asked the question that had been reverberating in her head for weeks.

'Mummy. Are you going to be okay?'

'Yes, I am.'

'So your arms and legs are okay too?'

'Yes, they'll be fine.' She looked at my bandages and, like her little sister before her, gently held out her tiny fingers and touched them. She stayed there for a quiet moment before slowly climbing up onto the end of my bed and dropping her sandals to the floor below.

As my health improved and the girls' acceptance of their new mum increased, we began venturing out as a family. First to the food court at the hospital, then to the local shops and finally to family gatherings. It was a gentle way for the girls to get used to people staring at us when they noticed I had nothing below the bandages covering my knees and elbows.

School holidays rolled around and with the zoo just down the road from the hospital, we decided to visit.

It was a gloriously sunny Melbourne day. Rod pushed my wheelchair through the crowds as the three girls bounced around me happily. The zoo was close to capacity, but the crowds parted as we rolled through. Every face bore a look of shock, and mothers hurriedly grabbed their children by the shoulders to make them look in the other direction.

'But, Mummy, what happened to that lady?' I heard over and over.

'Don't stare. Come on, let's look at the monkeys,' the parents responded.

We desperately tried to ignore people's reactions, but at

every turn we were the main attraction. The children were far more interested in looking at us than the animals, and a stabbing pain grew in my chest.

'Perhaps we should charge a fee and they can all just come and have a good look,' I growled at Rod as we arrived at the meerkat exhibit.

He hurried off to check on our girls, who had dashed off to play in the bushes behind the exhibit. As I waited for him to return, a young boy, about seven years old, came barrelling around the corner and almost landed in my lap. Pulling himself up, he looked me up and down.

'Hello,' he said happily. 'My name's Jack.'

'Hello, Jack,' I replied. 'My name's Mandy.'

'I'm here with my dad. I really like the meerkats.' He paused and then asked, 'Can I ask you what happened to your arms and legs?'

Taking a deep breath, I unclenched my jaw and began. 'Well, I got really sick and had to have my hands and feet chopped off.'

'Really? Why?'

'They died, and if they didn't go then I would have died too.'

'Did it hurt?'

'No.'

'Did they use a big knife?'

'Yes, I suppose they did. But I didn't feel anything because they made me go to sleep.'

'Oh, okay.' And with that, Jack was off.

Rod returned and sat next to me, and before I could tell him about the encounter, I heard Jack yelling. 'Dad! *Dad!* You've got to come and see this!' Jack came back round the corner, this time dragging his father behind him. 'Dad, come and see this lady.'

Jack's father's face filled with shock when he saw me, and instantly he began apologising and turning his son away.

'But, Dad, she's had her arms and legs chopped off!' Jack protested.

As Rod and I watched on, the two of them began pulling each other in opposite directions.

I interjected, calling out, 'It's okay, let him show you. He was incredibly polite just now – besides, if you don't, you'll never hear the end of it.'

Jack's dad smiled and visibly relaxed a little. He let his son explain what had happened to me. When Jack was finished, he gently took his arm. 'Thanks very much. You're right, we will be talking about you for the rest of the night.' As the two of them walked away, I could hear Jack continuing to explain my story over and over again.

'Are you okay with that?' Rod asked.

'Yeah, it's fine. At least he was kind enough to stop and talk to me. But I think I've had enough now. Can we head back?' I was emotionally and physically exhausted.

*

Back home, word had spread around the whole town. Until I got sick, Rod had been a teacher at our local college. Teaching was his life. Rod grieved the loss of his career, but committed to his new role as stay-at-home dad one hundred per cent. He cooked, cleaned, ironed uniforms, tied ponytails and explained what periods were. He paid the bills, shopped for groceries and helped with homework. Some women congratulated him for stepping up, commenting that their husbands would not have been as capable.

When I returned home, our roles shifted in another way. Now the kids helped me get dressed, pulled up my undies after I went to the toilet and put my hair up in ponytails. In the months that followed, the three girls became very comfortable taking my prosthetic hands and legs on or off as required.

But no one else in town had had a chance to get used to me. When I arrived back at the school car park for the first time, I was met with many shocked faces.

'Your mum's a pirate! Your mum's a robot!' Isobel cried furiously one night as she repeated what the kids at school had been saying. After a week of tears, it was obvious something needed to change.

I rang Issy's teacher and arranged for all the Grade 1 kids to be brought together for show and tell. Issy stood next to my wheelchair at the front of the room. Once they'd quietened down, I got straight to the point.

'Back in August I got really sick with a nasty bug that got into my blood. It's nothing to worry about, you can't catch it, but the only way I could stay alive was to have my hands and feet amputated.' Wide eyes watched as I raised my new plastic arm. 'Go on, honey, pull it off.'

Isobel grabbed my prosthetic hand and with a little twist, off it came. 'Wow!' The kids were amazed. They'd never seen anything like it.

'Issy, why don't you explain to everyone how my hands work?'

She held up my robotic hand and in a loud voice explained how the hand opened and closed. 'It has an electrode inside that picks up the electrical impulses from Mummy's arm.' She recited word for word the details I gave whenever I had to explain this anew. 'See – and if you touch the other side, it closes.'

Issy passed the hand around the room. Next were my legs. Again, she pulled my prosthetics off and showed everyone how they worked.

Hands shot up as tiny kids burst with questions.

'Did it hurt?'

'How big was the knife?'

'Did they use a chainsaw?'

'Can you feel through your plastic fingers?'

'Are you a pirate?'

For the next twenty minutes, nothing was out of bounds.

Then, as I told them how my tummy was cut open to take out all the yucky stuff the sepsis had left behind, a little boy stood up. 'I've got a scar too!' Lifting up his school shirt, he pointed to the long red line running through his belly button. 'The doctors put me to sleep too.'

*

That afternoon, as Rod pushed my wheelchair across the schoolyard, instead of pointing and hiding behind their mums, kids rushed over to me and Isobel to say hello. And they ran off eager to tell their mothers about my cool pirate legs and robot arms.

Now, years later, I am just a regular parent in the schoolyard. I don't get looks as I arrive. I no longer have conversations about how my hands work and my girls don't have to retell the story of what happened to me. I am just Mandy, another mum in the playground.

*

It's been eight years since I got sick. My daughters are teenagers now. It took me a long time to adjust to the new family dynamic, and many aspects will always be hard. My disability prevents us from doing many things we used to take for granted. I will never see the view from our local hilltop again and Rod and the girls choose not to hike there anymore since I can't go with them.

But I'm as busy as I ever was. I volunteer helping other quad amputees adjust to their new lives and giving talks at school. I'm working at the ABC sharing stories about people with disabilities and how we can live vibrant, rewarding lives.

So when the girls leave me behind to climb a set of steep stairs, I always ask them to take a photo of what's at the top. Then, on their return, I enjoy the few minutes we have when they describe to me what they saw. While I can't do what an able-bodied parent can, I can be present for my daughters – and I can show them how to face life's challenges with grace and an open mind.

* * *

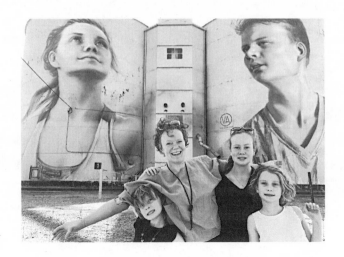

At thirty-nine years old, stay-at-home mum **Mandy McCracken** lost her hands and feet to sepsis, turning her world completely upside down. Now as a speaker, writer and Regional Storyteller Scholarship recipient at the ABC, Mandy is celebrating how living with a disability can be as vibrant as it is challenging.

Brian Edwards

from an interview with Eliza Hull

I was only eighteen when my partner announced she was pregnant. I felt both excited and nervous – a mixture of emotions. I was ready for the adventure that lay ahead. Yet suddenly my focus began to shift . As I eagerly awaited my baby's arrival, I was diagnosed with keratoconus, a condition which occurs when your cornea – the clear, dome-shaped front surface of your eye – thins and gradually bulges outwards into a cone shape. I was scared, fighting to stay well enough to be there for the birth of my child.

Bit by bit, my sight deteriorated. The doctors told me I had a brain tumour the size of a cricket ball. I'm a huge cricket fan, so this visual reference has always stuck in my mind. While I knew my sight would diminish, I held onto hope that it would one day fully return. I gripped onto my old life tightly, protecting it with all my might.

When my son Kodah was born, the midwife brought him over to me to hold. He reached up and touched me gently on the nose. I looked down and our eyes met. He had huge, blue eyes like pools of crystal-clear water. I still vividly remember them, and how he looked up at me when he hit me on the nose, as if to say, 'Dad, look! I'm down here.'

For the first three months of Kodah's life, I could see him. I got to watch his face and his body change and grow. But as the days went on, he became blurrier and blurrier – until I couldn't see him at all. I became completely blind and my sight has never returned.

It was a shock, because I always thought I'd recover my sight somehow. I never expected to be a blind dad. It was hard to adjust and let go of the life I knew as a sighted man. I dreamt of walking along the beach with my kids, swimming, playing football ... It hit me hard. All these ideas of what I thought parenting would and should look like vanished. I had to come to terms with the fact that parenting was going to be different for me.

By the time Kodah was five months old, I got so low I tried to commit suicide. I was very young, only eighteen, and struggling with my new identity. Hitting rock bottom like that taught me something; I promised myself I would never get that low again. I came to realise it's better to be here for my children.

After Kodah, we had a baby girl – Harlei – and then another baby girl, Rivah. I have never seen Harlei or Rivah. When my partner was pregnant with Harlei, I was scared of how I would cope not seeing her. I really struggled to accept myself and always focused on what I was missing out on instead of what I had. I thought that because I couldn't see my children I would love them differently. I used to second-guess myself a lot like that. But, if anything, not seeing them has actually brought me closer to them. They're everything to me, and I hope I am everything to them. I give them so much love and am a great, present father.

In my mind I have a visual of each of them. I used to sit there when they were babies and ask my partner to describe certain things about them to me. As I read them their bedtime stories and tucked them in, I would touch their nose and chin and get a visual in my mind of what they look like.

As you lose one sense, the others tend to pick up, but my sense of smell never got stronger, only my hearing. For this reason changing nappies was hard . I had to do it all by touch. The early years were challenging. Making up bottles was particularly difficult. When the baby was crying, I couldn't move as quickly as I wanted to. Luckily, they have come up with a bottle-making machine that allows you to pre-save your settings. It tops the formula up and puts the right amount of water in.

When my kids were young, I was very cautious. I didn't take them out unless I had support. I always needed my partner, mother or brother with me. With them to support me, I felt safe with my children out in the community. I occasionally wore one of the kids in a baby carrier, but I was always worried I was going to trip and fall on them, so I only ever did that when I had to. To be honest, we caught a lot of taxis, so in the end we did a limited amount of walking together.

My son was a late talker. At two he couldn't really talk; if he wanted something, he would simply point to it. But I obviously couldn't see that, so it was a lot harder for me to communicate and interact with him.

On one particular day I had my cane and I asked him, 'Do you want to go to the park?' I could hear him stomping his feet: he was all excited, running around buzzing like a bee. He then ran and got my shoes, put them in front of me and said matter-of-factly, 'Shoes.' I realised in that moment that he knew I couldn't see.

When my three-year-old daughter, Harlei, wants something, she knows she has to come and grab my hand and walk me towards it. Lately she's been walking me over to the fridge as she says 'Milk' or 'Juice.' It's incredible how kids adapt.

My children are still young. They know Dad can't see, but it's normal to them. My eldest, who is now ten, is asking more questions though, and sometimes he says he wishes I could see. He sees other parents at school and how the dads interact with their children. It doesn't mean he loves me any less, but he watches his friends kicking a ball with their fathers and he naturally compares it to our relationship. I just reassure him: Dad is still here, Dad still loves you. I just do things a bit differently, that's all.

Through having a disability, I have shown my children that having barriers in your life doesn't mean you have to be held back. I show them you can strive for whatever you set your mind on. They treat people with disabilities with respect, because they have a greater understanding and awareness of diversity in all its forms.

We are also Aboriginal. I am a Wiradjuri man. Both my parents are Aboriginal. My father passed away when I was nine, so I know what it's like to not have your dad around. This is one of the reasons I try to be as present as possible with my children.

My kids often say, 'We are not Aboriginal.' There are a lot of Indigenous kids at their school and there's a lot of stigma if you're fair – people say you're not really Aboriginal. I try to drum into my kids that it's not about skin colour. Their nan and pop are dark, but even so, my kids often don't feel Aboriginal.

I make sure we have representation of Indigenous and disabled people in our home, and I constantly keep the conversation going.

For me, I think a lot of the challenges come from outside the home, from broader society. A lot of people are so quick to jump to assumptions. They often say, 'Wow, you're a dad and you're blind!' I roll my eyes and say, 'Yes, and ..?' And then they respond, 'Wow that is amazing, you have three kids!' I have even had people ask, 'But how did you have them?' I just answer, 'Exactly the same way you had yours!' I say, 'I work, I own my own house and I do everything any other person does.' But they still say, 'Wow, you do all that and you're blind!' I think it's purely lack of education and lack of representation of people with disability.

I have been discriminated against, laughed at, stared at. Sometimes I'm not even allowed to eat in a restaurant with my family because I have my guide dog with me. All I am after is a family meal. I get so frustrated, but I try to stay calm and simply say, 'Okay, so you don't want my business?'

While society places continued challenges and barriers in the way of people with disability, I would tell any vision-impaired person wanting to have kids that anything is possible. You just have to go into it with an open mind. You also have to have patience; that's definitely key to successfully parenting with vision impairment.

For instance, when your baby is crying for a bottle, it might take you longer to find the bottle – so you need to be patient and stay calm. It's challenging, but rewarding at the same time.

You also have to have self-acceptance.

It's taken a long time to get there, but now I say I am a proud Aboriginal person with a disability. If I can empower someone by sharing my story, well, that's a real positive. Everyone says, 'Oh look at him, an Indigenous man with a disability who's a parent. He is so strong, he is so brave!' I like to be realistic. There have been some hard times for me, that's for sure. Some highs and some lows: that's just life. I adore my kids, though; they are my whole world. It took a long time to be comfortable with my new identity, but I owe it to them to be proud of who I am.

* * *

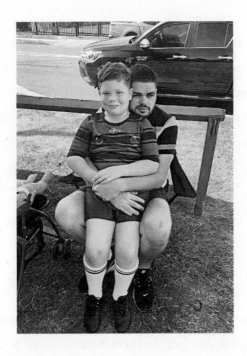

Brian Edwards is a proud Wiradjuri man and a disability advocate with Absec and the National Disability Insurance Scheme. Before becoming blind, he played rugby league for more than ten years with the Redfern All Blacks. Now he plays cricket with people who are blind. He is a DJ and has travelled the world performing.

Neangok Chair

from an interview with Eliza Hull

At just two months old, I acquired polio in Khartoum, in Sudan. I had a vaccination and the person who gave it to me was a student; unfortunately, they accidently put the needle into the muscle. The effects of this didn't show up straight away, but after a couple of days I had a fever and there was excruciating pain in my leg every time my mother tried to move it, so she rushed me straight back to hospital. The medical staff told her I had acquired polio, potentially as a result of the vaccine, and advised that I should use a walking frame to assist me as I learn to walk.

During those early years I struggled to move around, and my gait was uneven. When I was just two years old, medical professionals decided I should have major surgery; unfortunately, they made a mistake, cutting a vein and causing the muscles in my legs to deteriorate.

As a young child I had to use my hands to push my legs and feet to walk. In South Sudan, disability is not really something people feel proud about, but they accept it. My mother is a beautiful, humble person. I am one of eight children, but I am her special girl; she never rejected me or felt ashamed of my disability. Instead, she told me that nothing was wrong with me; she always made me feel included and accepted.

As I grew into a teenager, my disability began to affect my hips, knees and feet. Now my whole right leg is very weak.

In 2001, when I was just fifteen, the Second Sudanese Civil War escalated. I became displaced, but luckily I ended up finding one of my sister's friends, who told me we would need to leave immediately for Egypt. That trip was hot and hard, with lots of trains and travelling by van. My body ached but I had no other choice; I didn't want to be homeless. I needed to stay safe and protect my life.

When we arrived in Egypt, the United Nations accepted me as a refugee. But some weeks later, my sister's friend abandoned me. She had met a boyfriend who was able to take her with him to America; she left without telling me. At this point I had nowhere to go, nowhere to live, so the lady I was sharing a house with took me to the church for help. Luckily this woman had children and needed someone to take care of them. She was such a kind lady and trusted me with her kids. I felt privileged to have that opportunity. Her belief in me as a caregiver enabled me to see that being a parent was a possibility for me as a person with disability.

I was in Egypt for two years before my sister finally found me. She had been looking for me for years, she was asking around, trying to track me down but hadn't had any luck. I'll never forget the day we saw each other again; that was a very happy day; we hugged each other as tears streamed down my face. I was overwhelmed with relief and joy. We lived in Egypt together for five years, and then in 2006 we applied for refugee status in Australia and were accepted.

My sister had young children, so I was given another chance to look after kids. I was desperate for children of my own; I had always wanted kids, ever since I was a little girl. I always said I wanted to be a mother so that I could give them the love that my mother gave to me. I prayed and prayed that one day I would have children of my own.

At the age of thirty, ten years after I arrived in Australia, I fell pregnant with my first daughter. The pregnancy was extremely debilitating, mainly because I had severe morning sickness. I would spend one week in hospital, one week at home. My partner didn't take care of me, he didn't support me, I did everything myself. I had to take full responsibility. I am a strong woman, though – I've been through a lot and have had to be independent and fend for myself – so I just focused on the safe arrival of my child.

When I was getting close to full term, I struggled physically. I used a crutch to move around and I tried to rest as much as I could. The obstetrician told me that my hips were too small to birth the baby; I think he was scared for me to have a natural birth with my disability, so in the end I had a caesarean. I felt extremely sad, like my body had let me down. I really wanted to have the chance to have a natural birth, but it just wasn't possible.

In 2016, my beautiful daughter Breeana was born; she was everything I had hoped for and more. The early months were hard, though. I remember trying to carry her with a baby carrier while using my crutches; my body ached with every step. It was exhausting but I stayed positive because having her so close to me made everything feel worthwhile.

A year later I was pregnant again. I was very lucky to have my sister nearby to help me during the pregnancy, as it was challenging juggling a toddler and being pregnant.

After the birth of my second child, Billi, my husband and I broke up. Being a single mother has been extremely difficult, especially with a disability, but I have always been a very resilient person and focusing on my girls has kept me going when things have been really tough. At one stage my ex tried to take the children away from me, stating that I wasn't able to look after them due to my disability; he used it against me. Luckily, the Department of Health and Human Services gave me full custody of the children after months of fighting for them.

When Billi was just a baby, I would put her in the baby carrier to walk into town. I would use a crutch under one arm to support myself and then push the pram with Breeana in it with the other arm. It was a juggle! But I always kept a smile on my face because I felt incredibly lucky to have two beautiful girls who I love with all my heart. I felt blessed, so while the pain was heavy, they have made me feel light.

During those early years when the kids were young I faced a lot of discrimination. People were always staring at me, laughing, pointing, and looking me up and down. Sometimes when things got hard physically I asked for help, and sometimes people were rude and said no.

When I was juggling a pram and a baby carrier and my crutches, getting onto public transport was almost impossible, especially when the vehicle wasn't accessible and the driver wouldn't help me up. I don't drive, so it was our only means to get around the city. Often I would ask, 'I just need a hand to get up.' But he would scream, 'No, wait for the next tram.' Sometimes I wondered: is it because I am black? Is that why you will not help me and my children onto the tram? I try not to get too depressed; you just have to let it wash over you. If you sink into the discrimination you face for being a black person with a disability, you will be overcome by sadness.

To me, my disability is not something I ought to hide. People are always so curious and stop me on the street to ask what happened to my legs. People often assume I have had an accident because I use crutches. Often people feel sorry for me. They say, 'I'm so sorry that this has happened to you.' Others ask me questions, especially when I'm walking with my children. 'Oh, you've got two beautiful kids, but what happened to you?' 'Do you need help?' 'Are you okay?' 'How do you look after your kids?' Sometimes the voices get louder and louder, and more repetitive ; it can really affect me. I don't mind when people are curious and kind, but when people get pushy or make a joke it hurts deeply.

The most painful question I've been asked is: 'How could you bring kids into the world when you find it hard looking after yourself?' I wish I had answered by saying they have no idea what I can and can't do, but I was so shocked that instead I was silent.

I am proud. People may question my ability, but I'm an

incredible mother. I give my whole being to my children. I love them, take care of them, do everything for them. Yes, I move through the world differently and more slowly, but my house is full of love.

Sometimes it's really hard and I am absolutely exhausted. But when I see my kids smiling and running around calling me Mum, it's so beautiful. It's worth it no matter what.

Now as they continue to grow, they're often asking me questions, especially my younger one, she's very cheeky. She's always like, 'Mummy, can I ask you something?' I say, 'Of course.' She says, 'Mummy, what happened to your leg?' And I answer, 'I had polio when I was a baby.' I explain it to her, but she doesn't really understand. When she grows up, I will explain more of it. While they don't really understand, they know about my leg and they know that sometimes Mum is tired and in pain. I often turn to God when I'm in pain, because God gives me strength when times are challenging. I thank God that he blessed me with these beautiful children; they're my angels and for that I am forever thankful.

I hope to be able to teach my children not to judge a person with disability and to accept people for who they are. I want them to know that we are all the same. It doesn't matter if we are disabled or if we have a different skin colour. We are all human.

People with a disability are often told that we can't do things. To any other person with a disability thinking about having a child, I say: just do it. There is nothing that can stop you from having a beautiful family. I have one. Don't lose hope. Everything is okay: if I can do it, so can you.

* * *

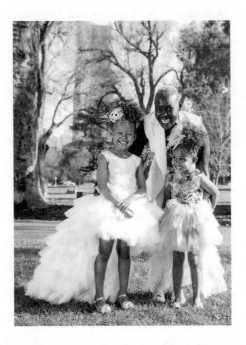

Neangok Chair is from South Sudan. She loves to listen to music, clean and cook. She dreams of one day being a doctor to support people with disability. Her main love is her two beautiful children.

Liel K. Bridgford

My aunt stood by the stove while my mum mixed the lettuce salad. They were discussing recipes, and Mum proudly exclaimed, '*Ze klum avoda!*' Being an excellent cook came naturally to her. Nothing was 'work'. They continued to exchange recipes throughout the evening. My cousins talked politics with my dad, and everyone asked me about primary school and what I wanted to be when I grew up. My sisters and I built a castle out of plastic disposable cups. We then indulged in the seven cakes my aunt had made, while my grandparents told us again how they escaped from the Nazis.

It was a regular Israeli family dinner. I was grateful to be living in Israel in the 2000s, rather than 1930s Europe when my grandparents grew up and were persecuted for their religion. Back then, children like me were murdered and tortured – I most likely would not have survived as a disabled Jewish kid. This knowledge hung over me like a dark cloud throughout my childhood.

*

I often wondered about how the little human inside me was developing. Would they have all their organs, bones, fingers, toes? Would they inherit my condition? These questions echoed in my brain throughout the pregnancy. And suddenly my body was on display for medical professionals again – to poke at, decide on, even slash open. I dreaded the familiar sensation of disembodiment – which I'd worked so hard to overcome – slipping back in. *Too bad I was born with ovaries and a vagina*, I thought. My body and records wouldn't be so exposed if I was the sperm provider in the mix. I envied my husband, who wore tidy suits to our appointments and drank full-strength coffee throughout the pregnancy. He didn't have to worry about his body's capacity to cope under the duress of pregnancy and birth. Such questions weighed heavily on my mind – how will my body respond to birth? How will I cope with parenting?

When I was growing up, there were always a lot of adults around – extended family or family friends. Everyone watched the children, and often relatives would feed, dress, comfort or entertain the kids. I spent many afternoons with my grandfather, playing noughts and crosses, cards or chess. My maternal grandmother was the *balabusta* of her city; containers filled with elaborate delicacies always filled her olive-skinned hands. My paternal grandmother was a poet and a Holocaust survivor, who cooked in small quantities but with great density. All the mother figures in my family seemed to manage childrearing and household work easily – it was their main realm, while the men did most of the paid work.

Everything in my family was big – the Jewish holidays, the

volume of political arguments, the reactions to another death in the streets of Gaza or Tel-Aviv. Everything except my disability, which was reduced to a 'problem' the doctors were working on via endless operations in which they'd break my bones and shove metal pins through them. Pins that then needed to shift to extend and straighten my leg. This trial-and-error process continued throughout my childhood. The doctors rarely discussed how my condition would manifest in adulthood or the ways in which my life was different to that of my peers. Their narrow focus was the lengths and angles of my limbs and joints.

*

At the thirteen-week scan I saw all the leg bones, and tears filled my eyes as a huge ball of anxiety melted in my chest.

*

I moved to Australia in my early twenties. By then I had completed military service and a university education and had met my fiancé. Moving to a safer, more accessible, more accepting country – where my partner had grown up – seemed like an easy decision. Australia, to me, was a place of freedom. I felt like Aladdin on the magic carpet. I could be whoever I desired, without the need to 'overcome' my disability. There were no wars here, no bombs exploding in cafés, and no one expected eighteen-year-olds to die for their country. All you had to do was chase your dreams – it was the perfect place to raise a family.

Arriving here was both disorienting and exhilarating. The feeling you got as a kid swirling on the carousel when the older kids pushed just a little too fast.

My excitement about Australia remained until I became a parent.

*

The first day or two were blissful. While I was physically exhausted, I was also overwhelmed by love and admiration for The Baby. He was already so different from me – so perfect. How was I going to be the perfect parent for him? Within days, the comments started piling on me – 'He's not latching properly.' 'Maybe it's the shape of your breasts.' 'Push him on while he's screaming.' 'Calm him down first.' Impossibly, I tried to follow every piece of contradictory and sometimes accusatory advice.

As I cared for our newborn, I secretly wondered how my body had created such perfection. I also wondered who I was now, and my mind chewed over these matters anxiously. Why could I not let go and be the relaxed mum I aspired to be? Why did my brain feel so heavy, empty and dark all at once? Now everyone called me 'Mum', as if I had automatically transformed into the template Australian Mother. I felt like a fraud – I couldn't breastfeed, I struggled with back and leg pain, and I couldn't meet the expectation that new mums walked the pram and the dog while holding a latté in a Keep Cup.

What previously felt like freedom now felt like a gaping hole. The magic carpet was shaky. Suddenly, when my leg was sore, I couldn't rest. The repetitive daily exercise routine which kept my pain at bay was gone – caring for a newborn left no time for it. Sleepless nights, breastfeeding and rocking a baby for hours were harder on my body than I had expected. Unlike the parenting I had experienced growing up, there weren't constantly other adults around. It was often just me, with a crying baby. And when I was in pain, it meant washing piled up and food stocks ran low. Even when my husband or other family members were there, I wanted to be an all-capable mother like those I grew up with – who in my memories seemed to have endless capacity for child -caring work. I wanted to be the best possible mother for my child, and I thought that meant being non-disabled. I thought I had to overcome my body. My understanding of attachment theory, together with my changed maternal brain, had led me to believe The Baby *needed* me to be everything, every minute of the day. Guilt flooded me if anyone else cared for The Baby, even my husband – The Baby's father. Suddenly I craved my mother's food, my sisters' reassuring voices and the way everyone thought of everybody else's needs constantly. I couldn't remember my parents struggling physically like I now did. I realised that even if they had struggled, they always had a familial, village-like network around them. Now, I was alone in a dark room in cold Melbourne, with a crying baby, a messy house and no village. Despite heavy pressure in my pelvis and searing back pain, I kept circling the little nursery rug, trying to settle The Baby. It often felt hopeless and dark. I didn't tell family members overseas how I was feeling because I knew they'd just worry or tell me to come back. This was home now, and I was determined to make it work.

As a new parent, I worked hard to hide or downplay my disability, as always. I liked to pretend it wasn't a part of me, but parenthood kept reminding me that it was. Very few people asked how I was managing the transition with my family across the ocean, and they usually followed up with misunderstandings or inaccessible suggestions. When I asked about settling The Baby, for instance, walking or rocking was the common advice. I nodded and swallowed down my truth. At every health check-up, I wondered whether my condition was mentioned in my file and hoped someone would ask. I was conflicted: I wanted it hidden, but I was desperate for support. No one asked.

From health professionals, books, apps and community members, I learnt there was one correct way to be an Australian Mother. This included exclusively breastfeeding for one year and cooking meals from scratch. One breastfeeding consultant told me to stop using nipple shields and pretend I was on a deserted island. I quickly got the message – here, any help was seen as cheating. I tried to live up to this woman-as-village fantasy. I pushed through sharp needle -like pain in my hip or knife-like pain in my foot because there was no one else to feed, change, settle or dress The Baby. I often ate only toast or cereal. My mother was mortified and gave me 'easy' recipes to follow. I could not admit to her that our definitions of easy were completely divergent. Empathising with my child was easy, but briefly standing over a hot stove was a struggle. Back home, I never had to explain this, because others would bring food over. Here, I was meant to change, educate, cook, clean, feed, do the laundry, host events, organise holidays, even send cards for Christian celebrations. I could ask for help – but only if I couldn't keep up and only for 'essential' support. A couple of friends and family members were occasionally able to assist. But when I accepted this help, it felt like a sign I was inferior. My internalised ableism screamed: *You're meant to manage all of this.* Despite enjoying watching my baby sleep, smile and learn, I felt I was failing to be a mother in the Jewish or Israeli model, and also failing to be an Australian Mother.

The anxiety that grew in pregnancy – the worry, rumination, self-doubt and racing heart – didn't disappear at birth. My baby was relatively happy, but when he was unsettled I felt it was a sign that I'd failed, despite intellectually knowing otherwise. And I missed my family. I imagined how different life would have been with them around. Only when I became a parent did I realise the unique ways my childhood village had held me. This village had both oppressed me and mitigated ableism. The same structures that told me I needed to be fixed advocated for the best education opportunities. The same people who told me to cover my leg, took care of my physical needs like they were their own. My village was like a loving-angry mother, shifting between rocking her baby and squeezing it too hard.

In Australia, I was suddenly both more and less disabled. Less disabled because attitudes here seemed to have progressed. More disabled because society expected new mothers to perform the work of an entire village. The first midwife I met told the class about 'Sideline Mums' and implied that if you couldn't participate in kids' sports, you were inadequate. Ableism does exist here; it just looks a little different.

I feared that if I told someone I was struggling, they wouldn't understand or help. Worst of all, I worried someone would mark my medical files, causing implications with social services or Australian immigration. My exacerbated pain or newfound anxiety were nothing anyone would understand. My heart sank as I read yet another Australian news story about a visa application being refused because of a disability. My exhausted brain tried to calculate my odds – *technically I have a disability, but does the government know? What if I need more support?* I was never sure my health records wouldn't influence the potential for me to stay in Australia permanently. And I couldn't risk the chance that my child would not have the life I'd wanted for him – away from missiles, safe rooms and mandatory service. Back home, as a male, he would eventually be recruited into the military, to fight a war I don't believe in.

My son was born four years after Lee was killed. Lee was a lively, musical person. He loved his family, the water, his friends and his country. He was my good friend's baby brother, and at only twenty was sent to Gaza to fight the continuation of our decades-old war. Lee's death left large holes in the hearts of my friend, her family and everyone they kn ew. I thought of this often as I tearily looked at my precious baby and imagined him serving in this deadly war at eighteen. I ached thinking of all the babies who had grown up only to be sent to die, because hatred was more popular than peace and due to the false notion that it was a privilege to sacrifice a life for our country. I thought of Asaf, with his kind, wide smile, who I served with in the Israeli Air Force. I recalled his funeral in the mountain cemetery, among the sad, thin trees. The soldiers I was a commander of at the time – his friends – coming to terms with his death. I didn't know how to console them. Asaf's mother seemed like she would break from the grief. These deaths and others – from all sides – were like dark skies over me that darkened further the moment my son was born. The grief and fear were endless and constant. I was desperate to protect my son.

I had to make parenting work in Australia. My pains were small sacrifices if they kept my child alive and allowed him to thrive in a country where his health and integrity mattered.

To deal with everything, I wrote and read. I was thirsty for understanding and connection. Someone recommended a book of stories by mothers. I devoured it and more of its kind. I cried, laughed and cleared some of the fog as I read – I wasn't the only one whose baby didn't gel with their boobs or who didn't feel like themselves since their child's birth.

Soon this wasn't enough, because none of the authors I read had a disability, or at least none revealed it. I wanted that part of me validated. I wanted it to be okay to be me. For the first time in my life, I read stories from others who have had similar experiences to mine, even though their bodies were entirely different. This revealed a new type of village, one I never knew existed. The disability community – where people openly and proudly shared their experiences, and advocated for justice. This village was founded on love and a strong belief in the value of each member. In this village everyone was equal and everyone held each other – although the holding was different from what I was used to. Instead of cooked meals, it was messages of understanding and care. Instead of rocking a baby, it was reading each other's words and believing. It was advocating for access so everyone can live their best life. This holding gave me courage to speak up and reach out.

I gradually learnt to trust people, as well as medical and social systems, despite the risks involved. I connected with others through stories, and it changed the way I viewed my disability and who I was as a person. I found a thread to hold my pieces together – my disabled identity. The fragmented pieces of myself seemed to work together like a beautiful, loud and bright collage. I no longer viewed myself as broken. Finding that thread has enabled me to let go of anxiety and find more joy within myself and with my child. I've learnt to watch him run and not feel guilty that I'm not joining in. I can say no to activities and know that he'll still have fun and learn from a day at home. I can shamelessly take my walking stick to the museum or the park.

My son is turning three soon, and I've learnt so much since the early days. I'm still disabled by attitudes and discrimination, but I'm working through my internalised ableism and on developing my self-affirmation. It has been challenging starting a village from scratch, but it has been easier than pretending I can function as an entire village myself. I've learnt that I must ask for help. I am building a village in ways my mother never had to. I'm using childcare as a pillar and readily accept offers of practical help, while working through the guilt that surfaces with that. I allow myself to rest while others bathe my child. My kid has learnt that riding a bike is a special Dad-time activity. My husband is now the main family cook, and we're both proud of that. I've stopped believing the ableist fantasy of mothers as the sole support for their child and realised there is no correct way to be a good parent. Trying to be a parent based on my family's model or the one represented in Australian mainstream culture didn't work. There is only the best way for me, my child and my family. Through trial and error, listening to my body, and through finding diverse, disabled role models, we're figuring out what this best way is.

Having the disability village helped me accept and celebrate who I am. But feeling comfortable and proud in my skin isn't a destination I've arrived at – it's a way of life I'm constantly working through. I still face the challenge of continuously re-defining what it means to be a good parent. Ableist expectations still come up occasionally – as self-judgements or feeling like a failure or imposter. I brush these off but the bitter taste in my mouth lingers. Continuously challenging what being a parent means is almost as tiring as caring for a newborn, but at least I get to sleep. With less anxiety about trying to be something I'm not, I've learn t to enjoy time with my child more and practi se mindfulness. Now, I celebrate that I am a unique parent with distinct skills and roles. I am the best parent for my child – good enough just as I am.

My kid has learnt so much from the fact that I am disabled. He has learnt about empathy: he regularly kisses my sore leg. He often helps other children around him when they're upset – fetching them tissues, patting, and asking how they're feeling. I believe that allowing space for feelings and accepting differences has helped him develop such qualities. I am sure he has benefit ted from the whole of me. It has taught him about self-love and resilience. We are both learning that disability and diversity are normal. I teach him about self-care when we exercise together and rest together. We are learning to balance caring for ourselves and each other simultaneously. He learns about giving back and reciprocal care, for example, when I volunteer at his day -care centre. We learn about justice, advocacy, inclusion, solidarity and accessibility. The clouds of our histories and the dark skies of current realities are still above us, but we search for the moon, smell the flowers and remind each other to notice and appreciate the little things. Over the years we have both learnt the various love and care languages we can use with people in our lives. Writing letters or messages, drawing a picture, buying a gift, helping a neighbour with gardening, or cuddling. I remind myself that cooking and other physical labour isn't the only way to show I care, and I practise gratitude. I am grateful for the village I grew up in, for the villages that we are constantly building, and for the disability pride that parenthood has allowed me to cultivate. This gift my child has given me is the most liberating of all. Embracing my truth and deciding to radically love and feel pride in all of myself has given me space for joy, creativity, laughter and a true bond with my child. I have all my villages to thank for this; the village I grew up in, the disability community village, and the villages of family – chosen and gifted. They are all my villages, and they all hold me up.

* * *

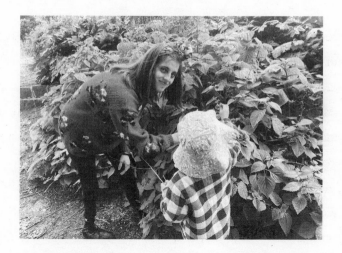

Liel K. Bridgford is a writer, poet, podcaster and a disability and justice advocate who is an ABC Top 5 Arts resident. Her work has been published by the ABC and in the *Spaced Zine* of The Waiting Room Arts Company. She works in the disability and mental health fields and identifies as a proud disabled, immigrant, non-conforming female.

Kristy Forbes

from an interview with Eliza Hull

I have four wonderful children; they're twenty-three, fifteen, ten and seven years old. They're all autistic – and so are my husband and I. As a family, we live our lives in a way that is aligned with neurodivergent identity, culture and lifestyle.

When I was pregnant seven years ago with my youngest, I was feeling happy and positive: my baby was on the way. I went to a regular check-up with a midwife, and she turned to me and said, 'Well, you wouldn't want to have any more children – that's enough for someone like you.'

I thought, *what the hell does that mean?* I couldn't get my head around it. Was she referring to the fact that my children are autistic? Did she think I didn't want to have any more autistic children? Then I realised she had said for someone like *you*: she was referring to the fact that I'm a disabled mother.

I'm proudly disabled; I have a really healthy sense of self. So when she said that, I thought, wow, you have no idea of the discrimination in what you've just said, how disempowering it is, and how potentially disconnecting that could be for a mother and child. You have made gross assumptions about my ability to parent based on the fact that I'm autistic. It's so hard to sustain a positive identity when the very people you're going to for support have attitudes like that. And they don't even realise how wrong it is.

I think these attitudes exist because we've been writing about autism in the same way for eighty years. Textbook autism is very different to real-life autism. The current diagnostic criteria for autism describe distressed or traumatised autistic people: they don't describe what an autistic person looks like when they're well supported, accommodated and understood. That's me. I'm an autistic person who, after forty-two years of struggle, now works diligently to support myself. I've worked hard to put together a toolkit and a network of supports. That, and I have a dose of privilege.

Most people wouldn't know I'm autistic until they see obvious signs, such as stimming or rocking. Medical professionals tend to subscribe to what's in the textbooks: they don't listen to the lived experience of autistic adults – there is a vast gulf between the autistic community and autism 'experts' (who are neurotypical).

I haven't always been proudly disabled, but having children has enabled me to navigate internalised ableism. I now challenge my thoughts. I pull myself up when I have those moments where I think *this is because I'm autistic* or *this is because I have ADHD*. I have my children in mind when I talk to myself like that. I have watched them go through things I went through at their age. My experience was completely different – I was rejected, abandoned, misunderstood and disapproved of. My children put things in perspective for me. Now I'm able to say to myself, 'If my child was facing this challenge, I would be encouraging them to have self-compassion and self-forgiveness. I would be reminding them that this is disability. It's not wilful or intentional behaviour. It's not laziness.'

My disability is not a small part of me. Some people separate themselves from their disability. But my disability, being autistic, is central to my being. It influences everything about me: my thoughts; my feelings; the way I process my environment; the food I choose; how I sleep; the way things feel, smell, look, taste and sound to me – and of course the way I parent. All of my life is influenced by disability.

Being an adult who is disabled means living in a society where you're constantly navigating other people's ableism. It's hard not to internalise that. When you feel like you're the only person who's experiencing ableism, it's isolating and lonely, so sometimes you blame yourself.

As a child I didn't know I was autistic. I just knew I was different. My experience of the world was far more expansive and involved than my peers. Sometimes they would look at me like, 'What are you talking about?' At school, I was put into isolation. I was always in conduct programs or behavioural modification programs. I didn't know there were reasons for that. I just thought I was inherently flawed or bad. The diagnostic criteria for autism and ADHD are based on the presentation in men, so a lot of women go undiagnosed.

Something that people don't talk about enough is that neurodivergence is hereditary. It's in our ancestry, it's genetic. When you understand autism not as a medical disorder but as an identity and a culture, you come to understand that sometimes we have co-occurring conditions as a result of not being supported properly in our lives. There can be intergenerational trauma in neurodivergent families. I came from a family where there was a lot of trauma: there was a lot of coping, but not really any nurturing. I don't blame anyone for that; it was just survival, and my family didn't have the understanding of neurodivergence that we have today. So when I didn't do the right thing, when I wasn't going about life the way people were expected to, I was blamed and reprimanded.

For a long time, I didn't realise that my children were autistic. But we got to the point where our family was in crisis. It's almost like we had to hit rock bottom in order for things to turn around. Our third child, who is now ten, is nonspeaking and requires significant, ongoing support. You could say that her autistic expression is textbook autism. It was undeniable and obvious, but when she was first diagnosed we didn't know our other children were autistic. We thought they were 'typical' because our 'typical' on both sides of the family was autism . It's very common for autistic people to have grown up in a particular family culture without realising it's autistic culture.

To begin with, having my child diagnosed was traumatic for me as a mother. I thought I was the worst person in the world to be raising a disabled child. How on earth was I going to be able to do it? Things got really dark, because I was fighting against it.

I thought, *I can cure this* and *This is my fault and I must fix it*. It makes me so sad to think about that now. I left my job to become a full-time carer. I was so stressed, but doing so meant it was just my baby and me. I would get on the floor and just be with her, tune in to her and observe. In doing so, I began to see things very differently to what we'd been told by the medical system. And I realised how disconnected I had become as a mother because of the medical understanding of my child. Medical professionals kept saying that her autism needed to be treated: this fed into my ideas about needing to fix and change her. Now, instead of turning to all the books by 'experts', I spent more time reading and listening to autistic adults. Very quickly, once I got a better understanding of autism, I realised that I too was autistic. I went through assessment and diagnosis, and then one by one each family member did. So it's been a really long process. Now that I know I'm autistic, I don't blame myself anymore. It didn't matter what kind of parent I was, my children would still have been autistic. And not only is that okay; it's wonderful.

I came to a place where I realised I was projecting my own trauma from not being understood as neurodivergent onto my children and their experiences. When I started to address what was unseen, unheard, unknown and invalidated within me, my children started to change. Our whole family began to transform, to explore what it mean s for us to be autistic, to live within autistic family culture. It's amazing how that happens. Now we absolutely embrace and celebrate our neurodivergent expressions. We are all different. We work together as a family to explore one another's support needs.

When the children are fighting or they're upset with each other, we always bring it back to: what is your sibling communicating with their body? Or we break it down: what's really going on here? We celebrate Autistic Pride Day and have ongoing conversations about what it means to be autistic. For us, it's now easy to celebrate who we are.

The greatest thing we have done as a family is immerse ourselves in the autistic community. By that, I mean other autistic parents and families. That's not something professionals will tell you to do, but it fundamentally changed our lives.

There is a lot of information about parenting that's perpetuated by the media, in GP waiting rooms, at the maternal and child health nurse centre, around what's healthy for our children and us. But when you're autistic, much of that stuff will *not* be healthy for you and your children. For example, many autistic people are introverted. We may have social anxiety. When our children go to kinder or school, that can be really hard for us as parents; we can be really anxious about being in spaces with other parents. Being in groups and spending time with lots of people is not healthy for us. We require a lot of downtime and we can become overwhelmed very easily. We can experience sensory overload very quickly. And then we can find ourselves in shutdown, meaning it's more challenging to look after our children and ourselves. Autistic people need to really explore what works for them and challenge what doesn't work – even if it's recommended by 'experts'.

As a family, we try not to have deadlines or fixed times in our routine that would cause pressure or panic. That's because we are also PDA. PDA is a particular expression of autism: it stands for pathological demand avoidance. I prefer to call it persistent drive for autonomy, a term coined by my friend and colleague Dr Wenn Lawson. Basically, it means we have heightened anxiety when anything threatens to compromise our autonomy. So we try to manage our daily life in a way that does not escalate anxiety. When we wake up in the morning, we're very casual about getting up and having food together. We are receptive, responsive and supportive of one another in terms of letting go of societal standards around what children should be achieving at a specific age. If my seven-year-old needs me to help her put pyjamas on, I'll do that and I won't shame her about it.

As a parent I have to put boundaries in place around my own needs as well. I have to explain to my children: 'I'm really struggling right now with the noise. So here's two things I can do. I can put my headphones on, and you can continue playing the keyboard. And that's okay. Or I won't put headphones on and you can continue making that noise, but what's going to happen is I'm going to be very overwhelmed; I'm going to be very grumpy.' That's not me threatening my children, it's me calmly explaining the process of what will happen so they can understand my choice. And they can relate to that, because it's their experience too. Reminding my children about autistic experience helps them understand the importance of me having space and allowing them to also have space when they need it. It models to them how to self-advocate.

My noise-cancelling headphones go on around five o'clock, because at that time of the day I've had all the noise, all the touching, all the talking I can handle. I don't have a sense of smell or taste anymore, thank goodness, because dinner would be a nightmare. Meals can be stressful for me, because I'm tactile-defensive. I don't like to touch wet things. Touching something that's cold and wet isn't just about a yucky feeling on my hand. It's a complete neurobiological response, a whole-body experience. I feel disgusting. I feel like I want to tear my skin off. I want to rage in response to some sensory inputs. But when you're a parent, you have to push through that stuff throughout the day, because there are times where you're the only person caring for your child. Changing nappies or cleaning up sick when your children are not well is just something you have to do. Sometimes I would sob over such things, and before I knew I was autistic I didn't understand why it was so hard for me.

My ten-year-old will grab a handful of flour and eat it, and then she'll cough and it will go all over the kitchen. I do have a good giggle over it, but I really struggle with food and crumbs and things like that being on the floor. I get very stressed out by it. My husband and I work really well together because there are things he can handle just fine that I can't, and there are things I can handle just fine that he can't. Now I realise I don't have to push through anymore. I can wear gloves!

Growing up, I was always told I should harden up. So I forced myself to do so. I was in such deep denial about my challenges when I came into adulthood that I wouldn't allow myself accommodations because I thought that was weakness. I would have pushed back at the idea of wearing gloves, headphones or really comfortable, loose-fitting clothing. But now as soon as I get home I get into the comfiest clothes I have. I have given myself permission to accommodate my needs.

There are times when if I have to do something I really struggle with, I find it helpful to have repetitive classical music in my headphones. Anything repetitive mimics stimming for me, so instead of rocking I can listen to something playing over and over. That has the same outcome for me on a neurobiological level.

Being able to say to one another, 'I can't talk right now' and not taking it personally is really important. We're not being rude or blunt or short; we're communicating like autistic folks. We don't have to mask inside our own home. Encouraging authenticity at home and being safe is vital for a family like ours.

We have spaces where we can jump on a mini trampoline or lie down. We can run up and jump on a crash pad. We have a sensory swing hanging from the roof. Music is also really important for us, so there's a drum kit and a piano. There are lots of outlets and opportunities for creative expression and lots of spaces to be alone. I make sure that at home I scream my heart out. I cut out time in my day to go out to the shed, put some really loud music on and move in whatever way I need to. I really understand that essential care for myself, in whatever form that takes, is a responsibility. Not a luxury. Because if I'm not engaging in autistic culture – which is stim movement, writing, music, all those things – if I'm not engaging with those things that bring me joy, my children don't get the best of me.

Our home is our safe space. It's a place where we all feel like we can be ourselves. It's going out in the community that can be challenging for us. We can never predict when we go out as a family whether it's going to be a great time or only last two minutes. So we always leave with radical acceptance around that, and for that reason we don't get to spend a lot of time out together. Instead, we have support workers who take each of our children out a couple of times a week in the afternoon to do something fun that won't be cut short because their siblings are not coping and they need to come home. My husband and I will go out with one of the children. Or we'll go out as a family but one of them will stay home if they choose. Once upon a time, I used to get really upset about that. But now, because I'm immersed in the autistic community and know other autistic parents, we understand that that's just normal for neurodivergent families. There's going to be one or two of us who can't handle going out today, or sometimes we will be out and we will become overwhelmed and we'll have to get out of there – and that's also okay.

I take my noise-cancelling headphones wherever I go. I don't necessarily always use them. If I'm in the city, I have to have them on to keep my threat response deescalated. My ten-year-old wears her headphones most of the day, everywhere she goes. We also have comfort items: lots of fidget tools that we take with us wherever we go.

I think the hardship for an autistic family is not that we're autistic. It's not the way we live. It's the lack of acceptance from the outside world, and the fear and frustration in knowing what our children will have to face. When most people have children, they don't have to think about preparing them to be discriminated against. When you're autistic, the chances that your children are also going to be autistic are pretty high. With my last baby, I was already thinking about the conversations we would have to have to prepare our child for the way they would be discriminated against in the world.

People said to us, 'You've got three autistic children. Why would you have another child?' That's the most horrendous thing for someone to say. They don't realise that what they're saying is, 'Your children are not whole and complete. Why would you have another one just like them?'

I refuse to modify my life, my hopes and dreams, or those of my children, to appease other people's discomfort. That would mean contributing to ignorance. My children are thriving and I am a happy mother. I feel a responsibility as an autistic adult to challenge the way we've been socially and culturally conditioned as a society.

Autistic parents experience huge amounts of self-doubt when they live in a world where all the support they access tells them that their parenting is inadequate and that their children are struggling because they're autistic. In fact, they're living in a society built on neuro-normative standards. It's not because of anything you as a parent are doing. Yet autistic parents are held responsible and shamed for their own disability, *and* for their children's disability. I refuse to be shamed. I had a fourth child knowing they'd be autistic like the rest of us, given our genetics.

Of course there are still moments when I am scared. Sometimes I still feel like I'm failing my children. I think that's a normal experience for any parent. But when we are autistic, we automatically hold ourselves responsible for anything that doesn't work out the way we think it should. We have to give ourselves permission to live out our hopes and dreams. We have the right to equity. We have the same right to quality of life as does any other human being. And if we want to have children, then there is an incredible, welcoming autistic community out there that can empower us to parent.

* * *

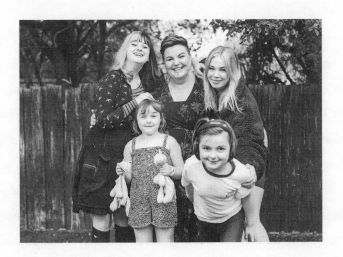

Kristy Forbes is an autistic parent to autistic children, and supports neurodivergent people and their families. She has an extensive background in education and now dedicates her time to training allied health professionals and creating supportive spaces for families raising neurodivergent children. She is also a Juris Doctor candidate focused on specialising in anti-discrimination law.

Shakira Hussein

My daughter started to describe me as *disabled* long before I was ready to do so myself. For several years after my diagnosis with remitting-relapsing multiple sclerosis, the most I was prepared to concede was that I had 'a potentially disabling disease', and having endured years of misdiagnosis and uncertainty, I wasn't entirely confident that even this much was true. Perhaps the neurologist who had dismissed the right-sided weakness that rendered me unable to walk without support as 'a psychiatric issue' would turn out to have been right after all, notwithstanding the MRI that had revealed lesions scattered across my brain, or the lumbar puncture that had detected inflation in my cerebro-spinal fluid. Anyway, even if I did have MS, I was undergoing treatment that would hopefully hold it in check. I was sometimes temporarily disabled, I might be permanently disabled at some undefined point in the future, I was self-injecting my prescribed medication on a daily basis in order to ward off disability. But I was not actually disabled – not yet.

Adalya didn't see the need for this type of tiptoeing around.

'I'm sick of the soft, caring voices,' she complained as our lives were flooded with healthcare professionals, support workers and counsellors in the wake of The Diagnosis, but she understood their basic message clearly enough. Her mother was *disabled* and she was a nine-year-old *young carer*. For which, read : guardian, defender, bodyguard.

Adalya's father had lived in Turkey since her early childhood, but we were very far from alone in the world. My brother and his wife lived around the corner from us in Canberra, my mother would fly down from Queensland to help out during moments of crisis, friends provided us with nourishing and delicious Indonesian, Malaysian and Lebanese meals. If we needed extra help, we only had to ask. But Adalya didn't believe that anyone else could look after me as well as she could. She certainly didn't trust me to look after myself.

Multiple sclerosis was not our only adversary. John Howard's government was determined to force single mothers to shift from welfare to work and to punish Muslims for our failure to uphold 'Australian values'. My PhD thesis on Muslim women and transnational feminism was years overdue for completion. The income I earned from tutoring and freelance writing was not enough to free us from dependence on Centrelink payments. *A disabled, brown-skinned, Muslim, welfare-dependent single mother sounds like a hate figure from an Andrew Bolt column*, I thought gloomily to myself. Although of course, I wasn't really disabled. Not yet.

*

When the MS was in remission, Adalya's caring responsibilities were relatively light. But during flares, she took charge of the household duties, from grocery shopping to meal preparation to washing up. And having taken control, she would decide that the entire system needed an overhaul and set about emptying cupboards, rearranging storage space, consulting the internet for advice on cooking techniques and cleaning hacks, as I lay on the sofa, immobilised by pain and fatigue. By the time the flares subsided, she had become extremely territorial over what she now regarded as 'her' domestic space and resisted any attempt to overturn her reforms.

'*That's not where the garam masala goes!*'

'Since when? It's always been—'

'Not anymore! I set up a new system!'

She was just as assertive when we were out and about. 'I'm her little walking stick!' she would announce, fending off anyone else who offered me physical assistance. And in fact, I did prefer to use my daughter's shoulder for support rather than be manhandled by whatever knight-in-shining-armour had decided to help out, as often as not by placing his hand on my bum.

'Adalya is very protective,' a friend commented.

'Only when it's my *mother*!' she retorted.

I didn't mind waiting in line to check in at airports (after all, I wasn't disabled), but Adalya would march up to the counter to explain that her mother had multiple sclerosis and was in need of special assistance during our travels. Even I found her equal parts endearing and annoying, and so far as the airline staff were concerned she was 100 per cent adorable. Such a grown-up, sensible little girl looking after her disabled, brown-skinned-and-therefore-presumably-non-English-speaking mother! There was nothing I could do but settle back in the airport wheelchair and glare in Muslim as Adalya explained my lunchbox cooler full of prefilled syringes to the security staff.

She would sit in the audience during forums on the 'the Muslim issue', quietly reading her book but ready to leap into action if required. 'Don't think that you can pick on my mother just because she's disabled! She's still got a daughter who can beat you up!' she intervened during one particularly fraught community meeting. Of course, we all just laughed fondly. That cute little girl wasn't strong enough to beat anyone up (and anyway, I wasn't really disabled).

Although, after more flares, another round of MRIs that showed new lesions and a recommendation from my neurologist to switch to more aggressive medication, I was eventually convinced that I did, in fact, have multiple sclerosis.

*

If there was a support group for parents whose offspring are excessively mature and responsible, I didn't know where to find it. And it wasn't a problem that got you much sympathy at the school gate. But I couldn't help feeling that Adalya was far too well-behaved for her own good. Her good conduct was a side effect of the multiple sclerosis and all the turmoil it had wrought. She simply couldn't afford to rock our family boat, for fear that it would sink to the bottom of the ocean. And she rebuffed offers of help from outsiders out of concern that our two-person household would be judged and found wanting.

'I don't want anyone to think that we're not coping,' she told me as she straightened out the living room.

'She'd rather clean the kitchen with her own tongue than let anyone else across the threshold to help,' I confided to friends. 'And other people have started taking advantage of her caring streak as well – neighbours, the parents of some of her friends. It's going to make her a magnet for every shitty male on the planet.'

Her plans for the future were built on the assumption that her role as my carer was only going to become more demanding over time. 'When I grow up, I want to have an interesting job, like a writer or an artist. Not just a job that makes a lot of money. But I want to earn enough money to be able to look after you.'

'Oh sweetheart, you're not going to have to look after me. I'll be okay.'

'Don't worry, I'm not going to spend all my money on you,' she reassured me. 'I'll need to save some of it for my own children.'

As touched as I was by this vision of Adalya as the breadwinner for me and my future grandchildren, I didn't want her life plans to be dominated by her role as a young carer. The multiple sclerosis had made a train wreck of my own career aspirations; I refused to let it blight hers as well. I tried to reset our relationship by telling her that while I was the captain of the household ship, she was my trustworthy First Mate. She did not take this demotion well.

'You talk to me as though I'm the bloody cabin boy!'

Mutiny was only avoided by acknowledging that I had overstepped the boundaries of my authority. How could I claim to be the captain, when I spent so much time below deck?

*

'Good anecdote, bad reality.' Carrie Fisher's words of wisdom had long been my talisman when dealing with difficult experiences, whether in the form of racism or misogyny or both. But multiple sclerosis was a bad reality that made for a fucking boring anecdote, so far as I was concerned. For the first time in my life, I was confronted by a difficult experience that I had absolutely no desire to write about. Most of what I'd read about disability was what Stella Young would later term 'inspiration porn'. I had no desire to write, let alone star in, that type of motivational feel-good story. Besides which, there were long periods of time when I was physically incapable of writing anything at all – when my vision was too blurred to read, my malfunctioning motor skills compromised my ability to type, when the vertigo was so severe that even turning my head on my pillow was enough to make me throw up and the pain was too all-consuming to allow space for coherent thought.

And once I'd recovered, there always seemed to be more urgent topics to write about than multiple sclerosis. My body had not been injured in a US drone attack on my family's village or poisoned by toxic chemicals due to negligence by a multinational corporation. It was just enduring friendly fire from the autoimmune system that was supposed to protect it. It hardly seemed important enough to be worth writing about. And anyway, I had a thesis to finish.

But as the multiple sclerosis occupied more and more of my time and attention, I began to recognise the parallels between ableism and my familiar territory of racism and sexism. While the multiple sclerosis was not an injustice in itself, I had experienced injustices during the long, bumpy, road to diagnosis and in the difficulties that I faced in obtaining timely support and treatment. Reading disabled writers like Harriet McBryde Johnson and Stella Young made me realise that it was possible to write about disability without indulging in inspiration porn. Which was convenient, as the continued onslaughts against my body meant that I could no longer kid myself that I wasn't really disabled.

Adalya had inherited my graphomania, filling notebook after notebook with (I assume) deep and meaningful thoughts. Emotional conversations would end with her stomping off to her bedroom, declaring 'another chapter for the tragi-comic coming of age memoir!' as she slammed the door behind her. I longed to read a sneak preview, but the hand-drawn snarling gargoyles on the notebook covers, alongside proclamations of PRIVATE, TOP SECRET and KEEP OUT, were enough to deter me.

But the realisation that she sometimes featured in my own published writing prompted her to go public with her own. She demanded right of reply to an article that I published after Julia Gillard became Australia's first female prime minister, in which I'd described Adalya as 'yelping about #historyinthemaking! as part of a bid for a #dayoffschool and a #triptoParliamentHouse'.

'You quoted things I said when I was asleep! You never quote things that make me sound awesome!'

She channelled her indignation into writing what the editor described as an 'out-of-the-mouths-of-babes thing' about the importance of compassion in politics and the lack of it in then Opposition leader Tony Abbott. Not bad for a first-timer, I thought. She certainly proved that she wasn't just using one of the most important events in Australia's political history as an excuse to skip school for the day.

I learnt my lesson from my mistake and was careful to obtain her consent when I was invited to contribute to an anthology about motherhood a few years later. However, by the time the proofs came through, she had long since forgotten that conversation.

'What the – I never gave you permission to write about this!'

'Yes, you did. You asked me whether it was a paid gig and when I said it was, you said "go for it!"'

'Look, I gotta say that does sound like you,' one of her friends agreed, and Adalya grudgingly conceded that it sounded like a plausible scenario. A scenario that once again provided her with the pretext to exercise her right of reply. 'Just another side of the story,' she told me as she sat down to write an essay for a youth literary journal about growing up with a mother with multiple sclerosis. At nineteen, she was ready to provide a public preview of the tragi-comic coming-of-age memoir we had joked about for so long.

I read it with a sense of trepidation. Of course, I had lived through the events she described, but that didn't make it any less difficult to read about them in my daughter's voice. Clearly I had failed in my attempts to quarantine her from the impact of multiple sclerosis. It had become as much a part of her identity as it is of mine. But I have no complaints about the thoughtful, generous and incidentally funny young woman who wrote that essay.

In some way, it feels as though every facet of my life has been shaped by my mother's health.

As her nerve cells were eroded by her body, I was built from the tools I tried to fix her with – tools forged from my mother's raw materials; her thirst for understanding, her front of fearlessness to everyone including herself.

*

Today Adalya's life has expanded: her concerns for my day-to-day welfare abated enough for her to move away from home to live with her partner. She was quick to reassure me that she would continue to be available to support me when required, living a short distance away in a home with an accessible bathroom and a ground floor bedroom for me to sleep in, if need be. I couldn't 'cure' her of her role as a young carer, any more than I could cure myself of disability. She has not so much grown out of that role as grown beyond it. And while I continue to make occasional cameo appearances in her writing as the comical, eccentric mother, she now publishes on topics ranging from music to art to women in science. The full-length version of her tragi-comic coming-of-age memoir remains unwritten ... so far as I know.

* * *

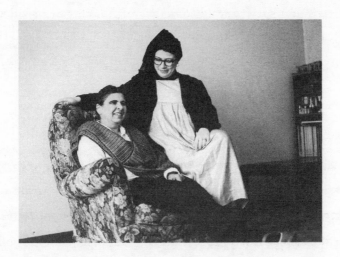

Shakira Hussein is a writer and researcher based at the University of Melbourne. She is the author of *From Victims to Suspects: Muslim women since 9/11* (Yale University Press/New South) and her work has been published in a wide range of academic, literary and media publications.

Rebekah G. Taussig

The night before our baby was born, I made my partner Micah take at least a hundred pictures of my full belly resting atop my paralysed legs and wheelchair. It was important to both of us to document this intersection of symbols – parenthood and disability. So often the two are imagined separately, as if they're a dichotomy – care receivers versus caregivers, drains on society versus contributors, diseased versus fertile. Everyone sorted tidily into boxes.

I would be lying if I said I'd always been able to imagine myself as a mum. I grew up in a body paralysed by a series of life-saving cancer treatments that tore through my tiny frame from the ages of one to three years old. Even as my body continued to grow into adolescence and young adulthood, there was no denying it was war-torn. I was monitored closely by many doctors, but not one of them seemed interested in talking with me about the possibility of conceiving, carrying, giving birth to or caring for a baby. 'We won't know until we know', I heard time and time again. Another way to put it might be, 'We'll cross that bridge when we are forced to.' But what if I was curious about the route we'd take to reach that bridge?

I was thirty-three when a nurse practitioner finally asked me if I wanted to have a baby. I was there for a routine exam, and she was covering appointments for the doctor I normally saw. I don't remember exactly how she worded it – 'Would you like to get pregnant?' or 'Are you and your partner planning to have kids?' – but I remember she asked it warmly and casually, and it surprised me. Is this how the conversation starts for non-disabled women? No medical professional had brought this question up with such unconcerned ease before. How empowering to be invited to consider! *Did* I want to have a baby?

'I've never really known if I *could* have a baby!' I said in a breathy rush.

'Well,' she said, surprised herself, 'let's find out!'

She connected me with other doctors in the hospital's high-risk pregnancy clinic, and just like that we were mapping out a route to the bridge so that we could decide for ourselves whether or not we wanted to cross it.

Despite several doctors giving us the green light to start trying, and although no one had ever given me a concrete reason why I couldn't or shouldn't get pregnant, I was shocked when that tiny test came back with two pink lines – positive! I should have been bursting with joy, but I actually felt full of anxiety and doubt. What did this mean? What was about to happen? Were we going to be okay? Before every appointment for at least the first twenty-five weeks, I was sure they'd tell me I'd lost the baby.

Each time I went to the bathroom, there was a part of me that expected to see pools of blood. If I didn't feel the baby kick for a stretch, I prepared myself for grieving. My body's deficiencies had been drilled so deeply into my mind that I could not fathom it being able to grow and protect a whole baby human. But it did – with very little drama.

As Micah and I thought through the options for our birth plan, my doctor connected me with a pelvic floor therapist. Her job was to perform an assessment so I could make decisions with more concrete information. Despite the widespread assumption that women with paralysis can't possibly push their babies out into the world, lots of them do. But I wanted to gather as much information as I possibly could before making a choice. Before we met in person, the therapist and I had a chat on the phone. She asked me a handful of questions about my abilities – How long can you stand? How do you pee? Describe how you push when you have a bowel movement. The questions were intimate and sometimes awkward, but I did my best to answer them for this stranger on the phone.

Then, abruptly, she said, 'You're not going to be able to do this.'

Instinctively, I pushed aside the punch of her words and asked, 'Why would that be? My doctor hasn't given me any indication that I *can't* give birth vaginally.'

Her answer was simple, and it didn't seem to have much to do with me at all. 'Look, I have worked with patients who are paralysed and patients who have given birth, and I just can't imagine that you'd be able to do it.'

'Okay, but have you ever worked with a paralysed woman who's given birth?'

'No, but I've worked with lots of paralysed women and lots of women who've given birth,' she repeated, as if that should mean something to me, 'and I can't fathom how you'll be able to do this.'

Her razor-sharp decisiveness took my breath away. The black-and-white authority she wielded on the subject directly contradicted everything my doctor had said, every bit of research I'd done on my own – and yet, in that moment, with her harsh voice ringing in my ears, I found myself feeling silly for assuming I could do this powerful act reserved for non-disabled mothers.

In retrospect, I wish I had pushed back instead of retreating. I wish I had asked if she'd read any literature on women with paralysis giving birth. Whether she knew that women in comas had given birth vaginally. But her voice was insistent and overwhelming; she simply could not imagine the intersection of these identities.

In the end, I did get a C-section. I agonised over the options, but we'd had a year of curveballs in other ways and ultimately I decided that a scheduled caesarean was the best choice. I would like to think that I came to this conclusion independently, that I was able to extract the ignorance of the pelvic floor therapist from my decision-making process. But I'll never really know how big a role it played subconsciously.

*

Culturally, we've inscribed so much meaning into the images of a pregnant belly and a visibly disabled body. The former is shorthand for life in abundance, while the latter is so often reduced to brokenness. And we seem to have very little experience seeing the two entwined. As this baby grew in my paralysed body, we busted through the tiny boxes allotted to us. It wasn't that I proved my body wasn't damaged – it very much is – but the brokenness and abundance folded into one another. As I splayed my fingers across my belly and felt our baby's lively kicks and rolls the night before he was born, I felt awe at our stubborn, sturdy defiance.

*

After Otto was born, I expected us to continue to defy the world's narrow expectations with as much ease as we did when he lived in my belly, and while I do believe our existence is in itself a sort of audacious subversion, I'm not sure how much of it I could describe as easy.

When he finally arrived, he shocked us with his knowing stares, his intense scowl, his loud and incessant screaming. I was enamoured with him, and also terrified of him. It was so easy to set him off and so difficult to calm him down. I expected that I would come into the role of his mother naturally and intuitively. And in some ways I guess I did. We figured out nursing like two champions. My boy has never struggled with eating. But I was devastated over and over again by my inability to soothe him the way his standing, bouncing, pacing dad could. I spent months trying to wrangle him into a wrap he could tolerate. There was at least a full week when he wouldn't even sit in my lap without howling. I wanted to be the living proof that disabled women could be mums too – *See? Look at us go!* But I felt profoundly incompetent. One night as Micah and I gave Otto a bath, I took a step back, looked at the two of them together, and thought – *they might be better off without me here.*

*

Slowly, oh so slowly, as the days melded into weeks, Otto and I got to know each other. I learnt how to read the signs that he needed a nap, and he learnt the textures and rhythms of my wheelchair; he started holding his fingers lightly against the tread on my wheels while I rolled him in soothing circles. And eventually – with time and a bit more sleep – I've started to recognise the sound of some familiar notes in this experience of parenting. In this realisation, I've discovered something jarring: parenting feels an awful lot like being disabled. How counterintuitive! I'd been taught that parenthood and disability were two separate, distinct experiences, and while my pregnancy invited me to play with the imagery, the act of parenting braided into the felt experience of disability in a breathtaking tangle of familiarity. It turns out my disabled body has actually given me the precise training I need to be Otto's mum. With time, parenting has started to feel more and more like hearing a cover of a song I've known by heart since I was a child.

*

My body and my baby are both unpredictable and take turns derailing our plans. They flourish when we lean into flexibility, imagination and adaptability. They require patience and endurance, attention and care – they thrive when we lean into interdependence. They inspire innovation and new ways of being together; they nurture a tender, sturdy intimacy in our family; they are bewildering, magical and demanding.

Disability and parenting have brought a host of limitations to the way we make (and break) plans, the venues we can (or, more often than not, can't) visit, the way it feels to look down a day (especially after a sleepless night). Running on empty, cancelling plans for a nap, doing extra research before we venture out – all of this was already part of the deal for me.

Like disability, parenting gives me immediate access to an insiders' club and fosters fast, deep bonds with people. I remember the morning I was on the phone with the doctor's office and the person on the other end of the line heard Otto fussing. I expected her to be annoyed, but she asked, 'Aww, how old? Is he teething? Oh, I know the feeling!' This brand of solidarity is something I've only known with other disabled people – the immediate relief that comes from being with someone who knows, really knows.

As Micah and I continued to make adaptations to our house and car to accommodate Otto's ever-evolving mobility, we relied on muscles that were already beefy from thinking creatively about how to make a new space accessible to me. We knew how important it was and how much patience it took to find the right tool. We tried so many bassinets, found a creative DIY arrangement for our crib, spent days researching high chairs, bouncy chairs and exersaucers, and tried at least four different wraps, all with the understanding that it would take time and be totally worth it.

Disability has prepared me perfectly for the inevitable moment at 2 am when I become convinced that my baby will never stop crying – that this single moment is the bubble I will live in for the rest of eternity, that I will never go out for drinks with friends again. I've had many moments when my back and legs reached peak pain – when I lost patience with my body for needing my attention – that felt like they'd stretch over the rest of time. But my body has taught me that nothing lasts forever. Even when everything stays the same, the light shifts and the story takes on a different tone. Otto brings me to this moment often, and when the familiar feeling starts to pop its head up, I know to say, 'Hello, old friend! I've been expecting you.' My disabled body and my growing baby remind me that none of this lasts forever – not the good or the bad, the hard nights or the best mornings.

Maybe more than anything else, disability has prepared me for the both/and experience of parenthood. More than any other experiences I've known, they've both brought profound depth, pain, joy, loss, connection, frustration and laughter to my life. They both make my heart ache and fill me with pride. They both bring days that make me want to quit the whole damn thing and days where all the stars align. Feeling loss does not negate gratitude. Feeling frustration doesn't diminish joy.

How interesting, to sit at the intersection between disability and parenting and feel the similarities wash over me again and again. Because not only are disability and parenting often imagined as two incompatible experiences, but parenthood is generally portrayed as a net gain and disability as an unequivocal loss. Even as both experiences are complicated and all-encompassing, isn't it interesting to see them pulled apart and pushed into such opposing categories? Can you imagine if the overwhelming response to new parents was heartbreak, condolences and pity? Or if culturally we were able to recognise potential value in disability? Can you imagine if we responded to parenthood and disability with a resounding, 'That could mean anything on earth to you! How do you feel today?' Can you imagine if disabled people were seen as viable, competent parents?

These experiences aren't a one-to-one comparison, and they aren't interchangeable. The experience of disability doesn't mean you automatically understand parenting, or vice versa. Obviously not. But I think we will all benefit if we open our narratives surrounding each. Parenthood can tangle with grief and loss. Disability can include joy and abundance. And goddammit – disabled parents exist. We get to be both. We always get to be both.

* * *

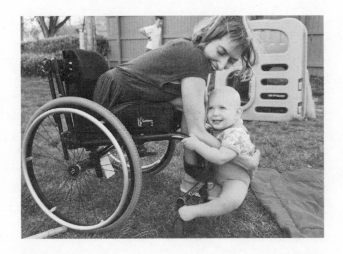

Rebekah Taussig is a Kansas City writer, educator and consultant, with a PhD in creative nonfiction and disability studies. She writes about the nuanced experience of disability on her Instagram, @sitting_pretty, and in her book *Sitting Pretty: The View from My Ordinary Resilient Disabled Body* and has been published in *Time* magazine.